EAT BETTER, FEEL BETTER

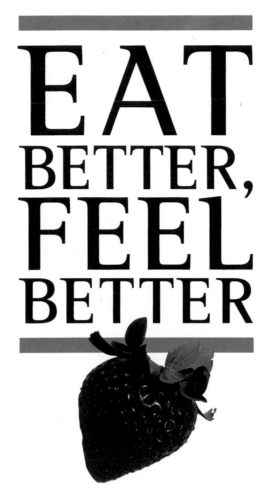

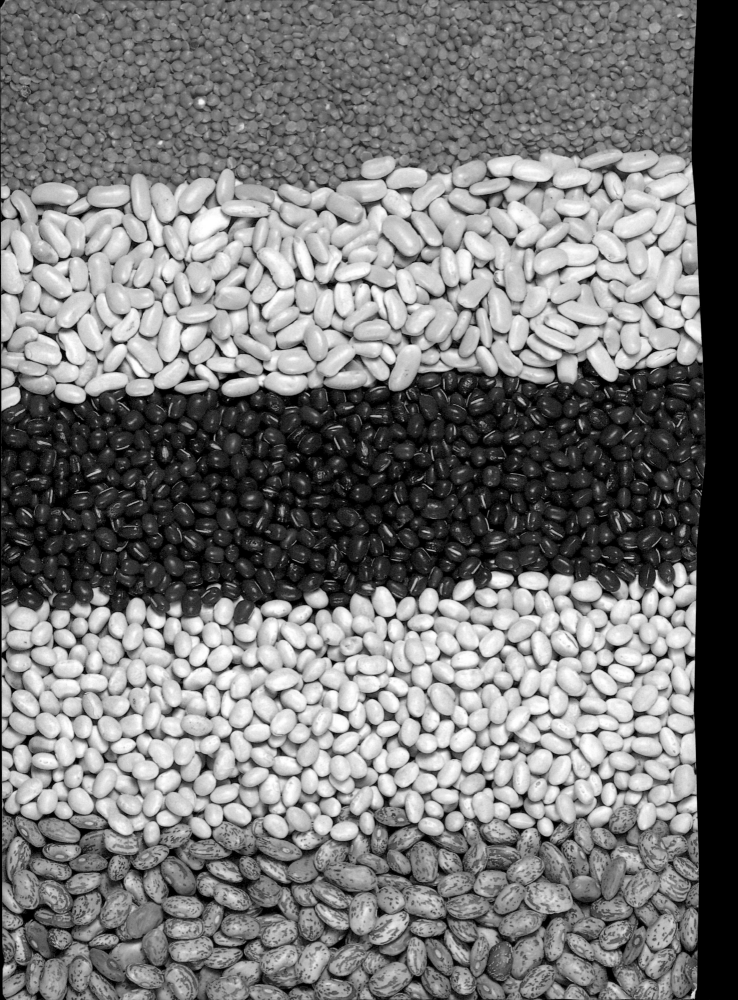

EAT BETTER, FEEL BETTER

*A visual directory of foods
and the nutrients they contain, plus a unique
section on combating common ailments*

Mary Deirdre Donovan
with
Consultant Nutrition Editors
Fiona Wilcock and Angela Dowden

A ☰ People's Medical Society® BOOK

A QUARTO BOOK

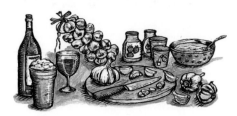

This book was designed and produced by
Quarto Publishing plc
The Old Brewery
6 Blundell Street
London, N7 9BH

Library of Congress Cataloging-in-Publication Data
Donovan, Mary Deirdre, 1955–
    Eat better, feel better: a visual directory of foods and the
nutrients they contain, plus a unique section on combating common
ailments / Mary Deirdre Donovan; with consultant nutrition editors
Fiona Wilcock and Angela Dowden.
       p. cm.
    Includes index.
    ISBN 1-882606-68-X (hbk.)–ISBN 1-882606-28-0 (pbk.)
    1. Nutrition. 2. Health. I. Title
RA784.D64 1998
613.2–dc21   97-32143
                                                CIP

The People's Medical Society is a nonprofit consumer health organization dedicated
to the principles of better, more responsive and less expensive medical care.
Organized in 1983, the People's Medical Society puts previously unavailable medical information
into the hands of consumers so that they can make informed decisions
about their own health care.

Membership in the People's Medical Society is $20 a year and includes a subscription
to the *People's Medical Society Newsletter*.

People's Medical Society
462 Walnut Street
Allentown, PA 18102, USA
Tel: 610-770-1670

Typeset by Genesis Typesetting and Central Southern Typesetters, Great Britain
Manufactured by Eray Scan Pte Ltd, Singapore
Printed by Leefung-Asco Printers Ltd, China

CONTENTS

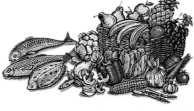

INTRODUCTION
8 – 21

FOODS
22 – 103

Vegetables 24

Fruits 42

Herbs 54

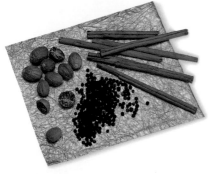

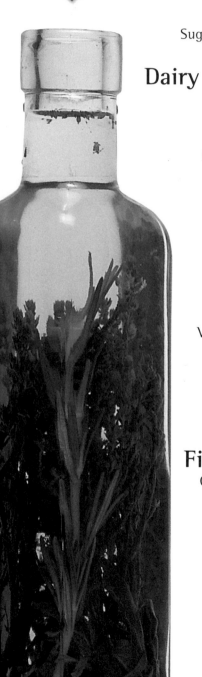

VITAMINS AND MINERALS
104 – 129

STAYING WELL WITH FOOD
130 – 153

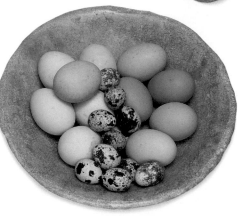

Why Do We Need To Look At Our Diet?

Over the last few decades more and more diseases have been linked to our dietary habits and the specific foods that we eat. We now know that, among other risk factors, poor diet is associated with heart disease, some cancers, obesity, hypertension, osteoporosis and anemia to name but a few diseases and ailments.

Surveys also show us that increasing numbers of meals as well as snacks are eaten away from the home, that we tend to graze throughout the day and that families rarely sit down to enjoy a meal together.

People also talk about the stresses of modern day living, coping with ever busier schedules and feeling unfit and unhealthy. Not surprisingly, all these things are linked, and our feeling of well-being is greatly influenced by what we eat. Frequent snacking on high-sugar and high-fat foods gives unhealthy peaks in blood sugar levels, leaves us short of essential vitamins and minerals and spoils the appetite for more nutritious foods. A diet containing plenty of fruits, vegetables and starchy foods such as grains and potatoes, with a moderate amount of dairy food and fish and a little meat once or twice a week promotes good health.

We need to look again at what we are eating and relearn how to eat to feel our best. This book will show you just how to do this by providing you with a clear guide to the essentials of a healthy diet, introducing you to major food ingredients and helping you match common health problems to your diet.

How to Eat a Healthy Diet

Nutrition experts have looked at the foods we eat and the diseases that afflict our societies and have come up with suggestions to optimize health.

Most of us need help to choose a healthy diet. Food guide pyramids and food grouping models do this by suggesting the type and proportion of foods we should eat for the best of health.

Food Pyramids and Plates

The Food Guide Pyramid devised by the United States Department of Agriculture (USDA) is a set of dietary recommendations that translates the suggested number of servings of various sorts of foods into a graphic image. The broad base of the pyramid includes breads, pasta, cereals, rice and other grains or foods made from grains. The majority of your daily food selections ought to come from this group. Fruits and vegetables make up the next layer. Dairy products such as milk, yogurt and cheeses are included on the same tier as meats, poultry, fish, eggs, beans and nuts. The top of the pyramid includes fats, oils and sweets, which should be eaten sparingly.

The Mediterranean Food Pyramid gives a strikingly similar message regarding the role of grains, fruits and vegetables. Some differences should be noted, however. Olive oil is considered important enough in the diet to deserve its own tier. Red meats occupy the top tier of the pyramid; it is suggested that they be consumed only a few times per month. Poultry and fish can be eaten a few times per week. Wine in moderation (one or two glasses a day) is an optional component of the diet.

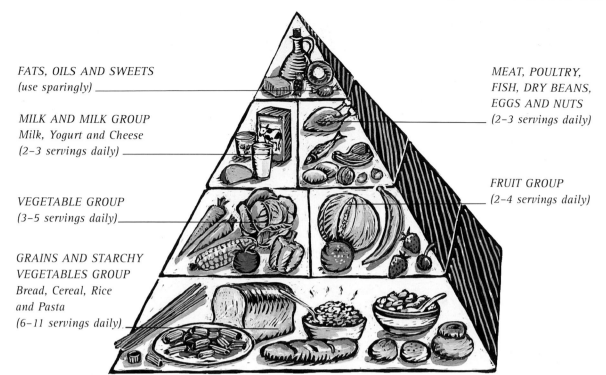

FATS, OILS AND SWEETS
(use sparingly)

MILK AND MILK GROUP
Milk, Yogurt and Cheese
(2–3 servings daily)

VEGETABLE GROUP
(3–5 servings daily)

GRAINS AND STARCHY
VEGETABLES GROUP
*Bread, Cereal, Rice
and Pasta
(6–11 servings daily)*

MEAT, POULTRY,
FISH, DRY BEANS,
EGGS AND NUTS
(2–3 servings daily)

FRUIT GROUP
(2–4 servings daily)

USDA FOOD GUIDE PYRAMID

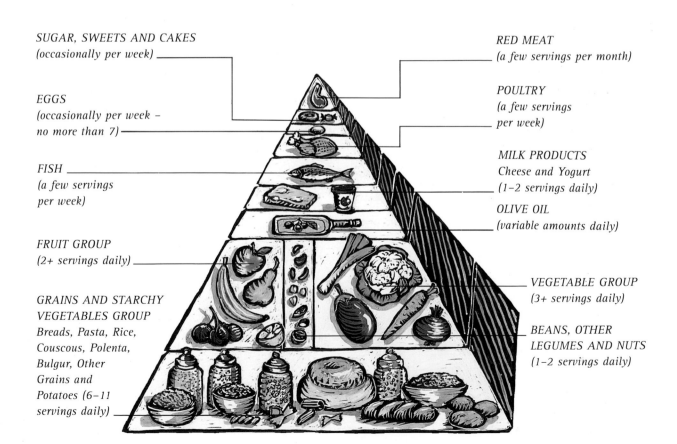

SUGAR, SWEETS AND CAKES
(occasionally per week)

EGGS
*(occasionally per week –
no more than 7)*

FISH
*(a few servings
per week)*

FRUIT GROUP
(2+ servings daily)

GRAINS AND STARCHY
VEGETABLES GROUP
*Breads, Pasta, Rice,
Couscous, Polenta,
Bulgur, Other
Grains and
Potatoes (6–11
servings daily)*

RED MEAT
(a few servings per month)

POULTRY
*(a few servings
per week)*

MILK PRODUCTS
*Cheese and Yogurt
(1–2 servings daily)*

OLIVE OIL
(variable amounts daily)

VEGETABLE GROUP
(3+ servings daily)

BEANS, OTHER
LEGUMES AND NUTS
(1–2 servings daily)

MEDITERRANEAN FOOD PYRAMID

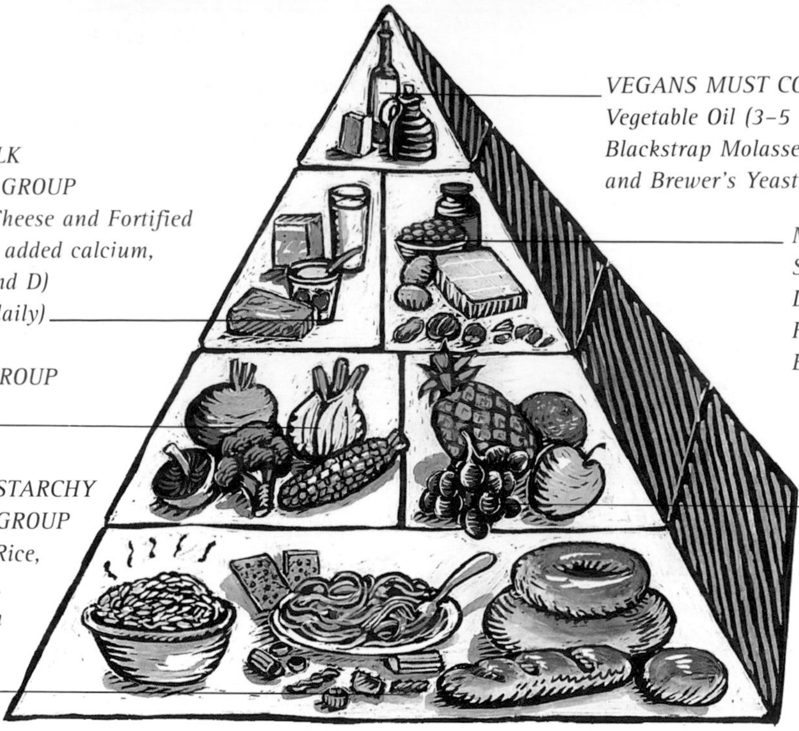

MILK AND MILK
SUBSTITUTES GROUP
Milk, Yogurt, Cheese and Fortified
Soy Milk (with added calcium,
vitamins B_{12} and D)
(2–4 servings daily)

VEGETABLE GROUP
(3+ servings)

GRAINS AND STARCHY
VEGETABLES GROUP
Bread, Cereal, Rice,
Pasta, Potatoes,
Corn and Green
Peas (6–11
servings)

VEGANS MUST CONSUME DAILY
Vegetable Oil (3–5 teaspoons),
Blackstrap Molasses (1 tablespoon)
and Brewer's Yeast (1 tablespoon)

MEAT AND FISH
SUBSTITUTES GROUP
Dry Beans, Nuts, Seeds,
Peanut Butter, Tofu and
Eggs (2–3 servings daily)

FRUIT GROUP
(2–4 servings)

VEGETARIAN FOOD PYRAMID

FRUIT AND
VEGETABLE GROUP
(5 servings daily)

MEAT, FISH AND
ALTERNATIVES
Poultry, Meat, Fish,
Eggs, Beans, Legumes
and Nuts (2–3 servings
per day)

GRAINS AND
STARCHY
VEGETABLES GROUP
Bread, Cereal and
Potatoes (5–11 servings
[e.g., a slice of bread]
daily)

MILK AND
DAIRY FOODS
Milk, Cheese and
Yogurt (2–3 servings
daily)

SUGAR, SWEETS
AND CAKES
(use sparingly)

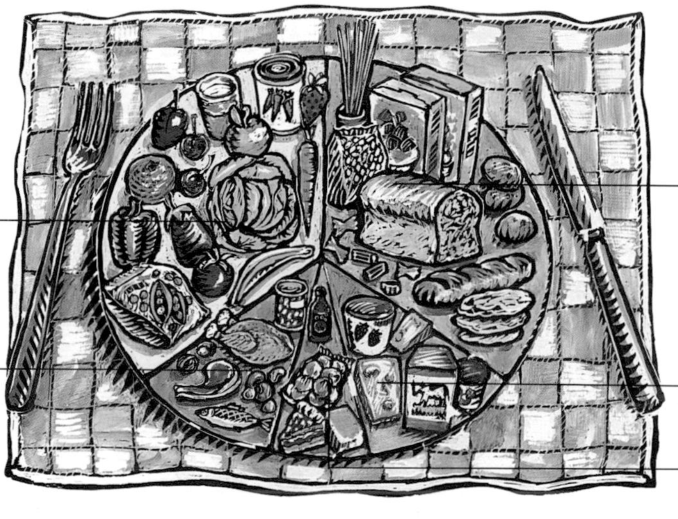

U.K. PLATE SYSTEM

The Vegetarian Food Pyramid gives the vegan option of replacing dairy products with milk substitutes such as soy or nut milks but suggests that they be fortified with calcium and vitamins B_{12} and D. (A vegan is a strict vegetarian who does not consume animal food or dairy products.) For those following a vegetarian diet meats, poultry, and fish can be replaced with dry beans, nuts, seeds, tofu, nut butters and eggs. The apex of this pyramid includes some foods that vegans must consume daily to maintain optimal levels of specific nutrients.

In the United Kingdom (U.K.) the "Balance of Good Health" uses a plate system rather than a pyramid, but the principle is the same. Two-thirds of the diet should be composed of fruit and vegetables (five servings a day), bread, other cereals and potatoes. The remaining third comprises milk and dairy foods, preferably low-fat; meat, fish and alternatives, also preferably low-fat versions; a small amount of foods containing fat, and a small amount of sugar.

WHAT THE FOOD GROUPS HAVE IN COMMON

Each food grouping model supports some basic principles. These are:

- maintaining a healthy body weight through a combination of a healthy diet and exercise
- thinking of a balanced diet as something to be achieved over the course of a day or week, rather than in each dish or meal
- keeping total fat intake at or below about 30 to 35 percent of the day's total calories
- replacing saturated fats with monounsaturated fats from sources such as olive oil
- drinking sufficient water throughout the day
- eating more fruits, vegetables and starchy foods, and selecting a good variety to produce energy and assure adequate levels of vitamins, minerals and fiber
- reducing the quantity of and frequency with which fatty meats, poultry, fish, eggs and whole milk cheeses are included in the diet
- reducing the amount of refined sugars consumed
- avoiding highly processed or refined foods
- keeping sodium consumption within a range of approximately 1,600 to 3,300 milligrams per day
- keeping alcohol consumption at moderate levels. (For women one or two glasses of wine a day, with one to two alcohol free days; for men slightly more.)*
- reducing the amount of dietary cholesterol in the diet (suggested by some models)
- For some people reducing total calorie intake

*Not all dietary recommendations condone alcohol or suggest that it is important or beneficial. This is an optional part of any diet.

What We Drink

Like vitamins and minerals, water is a noncalorific essential nutrient. It is needed to keep your body running properly. Our bodies are made primarily of water. Drinking the recommended eight glasses of water (53 fl oz/ 1.5 litres) per day keeps joints properly cushioned, helps to get the necessary nutrients to the spot where you need them and cleans out toxins from your system.

In moderation tea, coffee and other caffeinated beverages (especially colas) may not be harmful to most individuals; except for pregnant and breast- feeding women, three to five cups of coffee per day appear to have no adverse effects. However, those who become nervous or jittery or who have trouble sleeping should cut back or eliminate caffeine. Another option is to have only one caffeinated beverage, early in the day.

Alcoholic beverages are also deemed admissible in most healthy eating plans as long as there are no health indications such as liver conditions, diabetes, alcoholism and pregnancy that would make alcohol a problem. In fact, many studies have pointed to a correlation between moderate consumption of alcohol (and in particular wine) and a decreased incidence of heart disease.

Juices made from whole fruit and vegetables are usually calculated as part of your daily serving of vegetables. Juice drinks, as well as other soft drinks, on the other hand, are generally nothing more than sweetened, flavored water. Beware of any claims on the label maintaining that the beverage has 100 percent of the day's requirement for various vitamins and minerals anyway. If you are eating properly, you should be getting adequate supplies of vitamins and minerals anyway. If you aren't, the quantity of refined sugar you will be ingesting along with those calories makes their nutritional value suspect.

▼ *It's important to drink plenty throughout the day. Around eight glasses of fluid is the ideal to aim for, but avoid too many sugary drinks.*

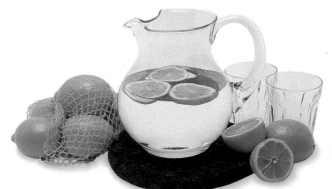

The Role of Exercise

A sedentary lifestyle is in part accountable for the huge increase in the numbers of people who are overweight and obese. It also affects the way many people feel at the end of the day. Instead of being physically tired, ready to enjoy a deep, rejuvenating sleep, we are left anxious, fretful and mentally tired. Our bodies are suffering from lack of aerobic, anaerobic and stretching exercise.

Exercise cannot be ignored as part of a daily routine. The many benefits include:

- weight loss
- improved muscle tone
- increased endurance
- freedom from insomnia
- prevention or delay in onset of osteoporosis
- reduction of severity of PMS and menstrual discomfort
- clearer thinking and better memory
- improved outlook on life in general

▼ *Exercises that work muscles through improving their strength (anaerobic exercise) and improving their flexibility (stretching) are as important as aerobic exercises.*

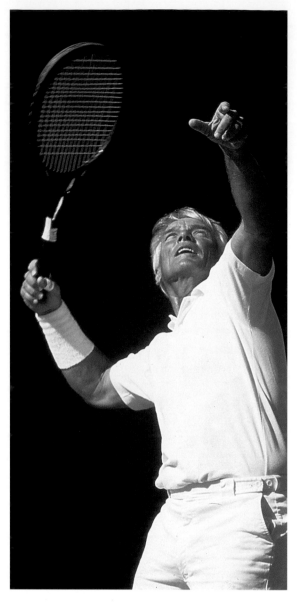

▲ *Including regular aerobic exercise in your weekly schedule is an important way to maintain a healthy heart and lungs. Choose whichever activity you enjoy most.*

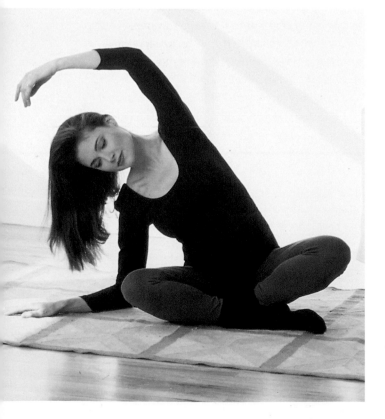

Aerobic activities are those that increase oxygen consumption and cause our cardiovascular system to work harder. Jogging, running, walking, tennis, soccer and swimming are all excellent options. Anaerobic activities do not increase oxygen consumption and mainly use large muscles. The types of exercise in this category include calisthenics, strength training, weight-lifting and resistance exercise. Stretching exercises include yoga and t'ai chi. The most effective exercise routines incorporate all three types of exercise over the course of a week.

What's In The Food We Eat?

All food provides us with energy, which is usually measured in calories (cal) or kilojoules (kJ). Energy is provided by carbohydrates and protein (4 cal per gram), fat (9 cal per gram) and alcohol (7 cal per gram). Although carbohydrates and protein both provide the same amount of calories, the body tends to use carbohydrates and fat for its main supply of energy. Because fat also makes food very palatable, it is easy to eat too much fat. Starchy foods such as bread, potatoes, rice and pasta contain little fat but lots of carbohydrates, so this is why we are encouraged to fill up on these sorts of foods.

Without energy we could not maintain life, but we need to balance the amount of energy we need against the amount we consume. If we eat a lot but don't exercise enough to use up the excess calories, then energy will be stored in the body as fat. Conversely, fat stores are used up when the amount of energy supplied in the diet doesn't match the amount required to maintain all the body processes and activity.

Some people count calories in order to help them maintain their weight, but it can be unhelpful to become too obsessive about counting every calorie.

With increasing numbers of people becoming overweight and obese, it is important to recognize the dual role of diet and exercise. Obesity leads to many chronic disease states including hypertension, heart disease, some cancers, diabetes and arthritis. Some emotional and psychological disorders are also linked to being overweight.

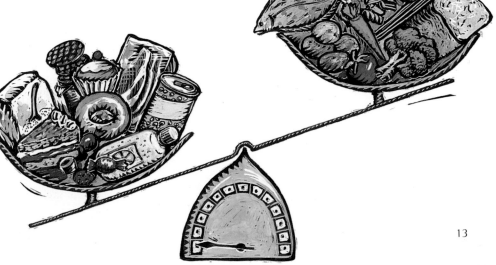

▶ *The key to a healthy diet is achieving balance. Cereals, fruit and vegetables should be eaten often, while high fat, high-sugar foods should only be eaten occasionally.*

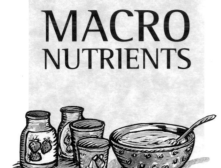

MACRO NUTRIENTS

Proteins, carbohydrates and fats are the major, or macro, nutrients in food.

Proteins

Few people ever suffer from protein deficiencies. Instead, our diets tend to include too much protein, especially meats. This has the effect of increasing the quantity of saturated fats in our diets, leading to high blood cholesterol levels.

Shifting toward leaner cuts of meat, and using more skinless poultry, fish and foods such as dried beans and tofu, will provide protein without too much fat.

Proteins are composed of smaller groups known as amino acids. Some can be made in the body while others must be provided in the diet. These are essential (or indispensable) amino acids (EAAs or IAAs).

Foods such as meat, milk, cheese and eggs are "complete" proteins. This means that these foods supply the essential amino acids in the correct amounts. In general, a single 6-ounce (175-gram) portion of meat, poultry or fish coupled with one to three servings of a low-fat dairy food throughout the day will meet an individual's requirements. For a vegetarian, about 10 ounces (250 grams) of beans or legumes are needed daily. Plant-based foods contain protein but may lack one or more EAAs (IAAs). This deficiency is usually overcome by eating different plant foods together; for example, legumes and grains, nuts and grains.

Most classic vegetarian meals rely on balanced food combinations such as rice and beans that provide all of the

essential amino acids (EAAs or IAAs) in good balance.

For a vegan more care is required, and nuts, and legumes should be eaten regularly.

Carbohydrates

There are two types of carbohydrates: starches and sugars. Complex carbohydrates contribute to a healthy diet by providing an energy source that is released in an even, gradual manner. Your body can use fats and protein to provide energy, but these nutrients must first be altered into a form that your body can use. Complex carbohydrates are the body's preferred energy source.

Starchy foods such as potatoes, bread, rice, pasta, noodles, corn and dried legumes provide not only carbohydrates but also fiber, protein, vitamins and minerals.

Sugars are found in milk as lactose and in fruits, vegetables and honey as fructose. Sucrose is usually obtained by extraction from sugar cane or beet and is the table sugar we know.

Sugars vary in their ability to cause dental decay, but all except lactose can be fermented by bacteria in the mouth, yielding acid that attacks the tooth enamel.

REFINED SUGARS

Food manufacturers sometimes use alternative names for sugars. These can include invert sugar or syrup, honey, raw sugar, brown sugar, cane sugar, muscavado sugar, molasses, concentrated fruit juice and maple syrup.

▼ *"Simple" sugars found in foods such as honey, jams, table sugar and fruit juice can cause tooth decay if eaten to excess.*

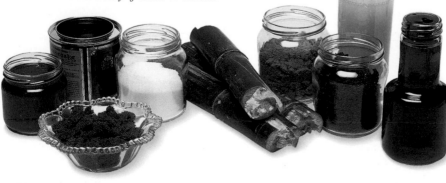

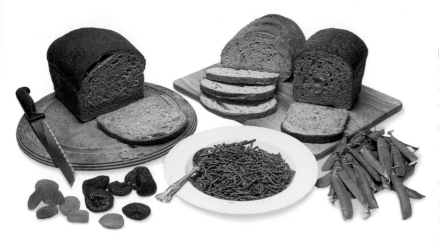

▲ *Carbohydrates are vital energy foods in our diets. Good sources include bread, cereals, legumes, fruits and vegetables.*

Glucose, dextrose, maltose and fructose are commonly used and are no different to sucrose sugar in their effect on the teeth.

Sugar can boost the caloric level of foods without offering any other nutritional benefit.

FIBER

Dietary fiber or nonstarch polysaccharides are only found in plant foods. Some are soluble and some insoluble but both play an important role in regulating the functioning of the intestines.

Fiber can hinder the absorption of some minerals from foods, but this may only be a significant problem to vegans who eat large quantities of beans and whole-grain cereals.

Some fiber is fermented in the large intestine and this provides a small amount of energy. There is evidence that diets rich in fiber help with diabetic control, and soluble fiber from oats, legumes and guar gum has also been shown to help lower blood cholesterol

levels. High-fiber diets are bulky, and this can aid calorie-controlled weight loss, constipation and some forms of irritable bowel syndrome.

Some sources of fiber include:

- **Good sources:** peas; beans; dried apricots and figs; whole wheat, grain, and rye breads; bran-based breakfast cereals
- **Fair sources:** fruits, vegetables and nuts; pasta

Meeting Carbohydrate and Fiber Requirements

Most dietary guidelines recommend that at least 50 percent of your day's total calories should come from carbohydrates, with as few of those calories as possible derived from refined sugars found in sweeteners, candies, pastries and carbonated beverages.

Fiber is another important part of a healthy diet. Most people don't include the correct level of fiber-rich foods in their diets. Four portions of fruits and vegetables and two cereal-based dishes will meet most people's requirements.

Fats and Oils

Fat is needed by the body to build cells, provide energy and to protect organs from damage. Vitamins A, D, E and K are dissolved in fat, and fat is needed for their absorption.

Fat is made up of two compounds, fatty acids and glycerol. The fatty acids may be saturated, monounsaturated or polyunsaturated, and different foods contain a mixture of each. Foods that contain a lot of saturated fatty acids include butter, cream, fatty meats, bacon fat, poultry skin and lard.

Saturated fatty acids raise the levels of undesirable low-density lipoprotein (LDL) cholesterol in the blood, and dietary recommendations are that no more than 10 percent of total calories should be provided by saturated fatty acids.

Conversely, mono-unsaturated fatty acids have a tendency to lower the levels of undesirable cholesterol in the blood and raise the level of more beneficial forms. The net result is that individuals whose diets rely upon mono-unsaturated fatty acids, rather than saturated fats, are less likely to develop hardening of the arteries (atherosclerosis). Olive and canola (rapeseed) oil contain mostly mono-unsaturated fatty acids, although nuts, avocado, meat and dairy products contain some too.

Polyunsaturated fats and oils are still preferred to saturated fats but do not have the same benefits as monoun-saturated fats. Polyunsaturated fats are found mainly in sunflower and corn oils and in some vegetables.

Vegetable oils are often used in the preparation of shortening and margarine. Part of the process is known as hydrogenation, which changes the overall structure of the fat. Substances called trans fatty acids are produced, and they are believed to behave in a similar way to saturated fatty acids.

Oily fish contain fatty acids called long chain polyunsaturates. People such as Inuits who eat a lot of oily fish are far less prone to heart disease and strokes. This is because the fatty acids make the blood "thinner" and less likely to clot.

Some people use supplements of these beneficial fatty acids. EPA (ecosapentaenoic acid) and DHA (docasahexaenoic acid) are the chief constituents.

CHOLESTEROL

Cholesterol is another type of fat. Dietary cholesterol is found in foods, particularly animal products. Blood or serum cholesterol is that which is found in your bloodstream and made in the liver.

Dietary cholesterol has a smaller effect on blood cholesterol than saturated fat. In most people the liver can alter the amount of blood cholesterol it makes according to how much dietary cholesterol is eaten.

Plant-based foods, even those high in saturated fats, do not contain cholesterol. This means that peanut butter, almonds, olives, beans and sesame seeds are all cholesterol-free.

Keeping Dietary Fat at a Healthy Level

The problem facing most people is that they consume too much fat; often 40 percent and more of the calories they eat comes from fat. It appears that as an individual's fat intake goes up, so does the risk of developing heart disease, stroke and hardening of the arteries.

Most nutritionists suggest that fat calories should be kept between 30 and 35 percent of the day's total calories.

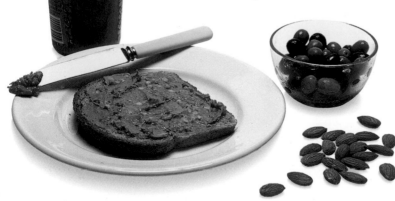

▲ *Some fat (for example, from vegetable oil and nuts) is essential in the diet, but too much—especially saturated fat—is undesirable.*

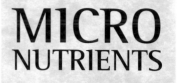
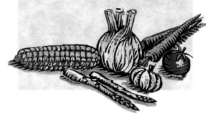

MICRO NUTRIENTS

Vitamins and Minerals

These micronutrients are vital for various functions in the human body.

Many folk cures were based on the fact that a specific food could replenish the missing nutrient. Around the turn of the twentieth century, chemists were able to isolate these compounds. They were initially identified by letters and later given more specific names. Deficiency diseases were also identified. National dietary recommendations for vitamins and minerals have been based on the levels required to prevent those diseases. (See pages 106–129 for more information about specific vitamins and minerals and their relationship to health and well-being.)

WATER-SOLUBLE VITAMINS

Vitamin C (ascorbic acid) and the B vitamins can be dissolved in water. This means that you need to replenish these vitamins daily, since they are readily lost from the body in waste fluids. They are also sensitive to prolonged exposure to heat, air and light. Cooking foods to retain maximum levels of the water-soluble vitamins is a challenge, but one that can be accomplished as long as you are careful not to overcook foods, prepare or cook them too far in advance or leave them in water.

FAT-SOLUBLE VITAMINS

Vitamins A, D, E and K are fat-soluble. This means that they are stored in fat, which is far less simple to remove from the body than water. *Megadoses* of vitamin supplements can easily cause toxic levels to build up, leading to serious disease, even death. Unlike water-soluble vitamins, these vitamins are usually stable during cooking.

ANTIOXIDANTS

Carotenes, including beta-carotene, as well as vitamin C and vitamin E and selenium, have antioxidant properties. This means they mop up free radicals that are produced by the body and that can attack important molecules such as DNA and proteins. If the DNA in a cell is damaged, the cell is more likely to become cancerous. Free radicals can also oxidize polyunsaturates in foods and cells and may alter the undesirable LDL blood cholesterol, leading to atherosclerosis, or hardening of the arteries.

Foods rich in carotenes, vitamin C and vitamin E appear to protect against this damage and include yellow and orange fruits and orange and dark-green vegetables.

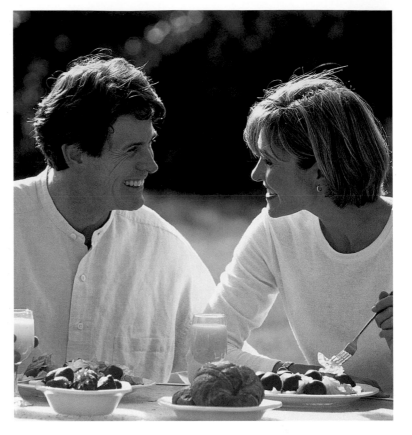

▲ *Micronutrients (vitamins and minerals needed only in small amounts by the body) are essential for good health and can be obtained by eating a diet rich in fresh foods.*

MAJOR MINERALS

Calcium, potassium, phosphorus, chloride, magnesium, zinc, iron and sodium are required by your body in significant quantities and need to be part of your daily diet.

TRACE MINERALS

Fluoride, copper, selenium, iodine, manganese, chromium and cobalt are also required but in tiny quantities.

Meeting Dietary Requirements for Vitamins and Minerals

Today, as we continue to learn more about the role of vitamins and minerals in maintaining health, questions about the value of supplementation are cropping up. Many people use vitamin and mineral supplements to bolster their immune systems and help prevent micronutrient deficiencies. Modest supplementation is perfectly safe, but self-medication can have serious consequences if an individual takes megadoses, especially of the fat-soluble vitamins and some minerals. (See also *Vitamins and Minerals* on pages 106–129.)

Vitamin and mineral supplementation should not be necessary if you don't have any special needs and follow a varied daily diet rich in whole grains, fruits, vegetables and low-fat dairy foods.

Creating a "Healthy" Diet Plan

Choosing foods from the various tiers of the relevant pyramid to make up our daily diet is a good way to be sure that we are getting a balanced assortment of all the nutrients we need. Relearning about food and adjusting our expectations and attitudes may take a while but are important in developing a successful "healthy" diet plan.

A variety of foods is one way to ensure that your meals are appealing, both in their appearance and their overall flavor. After all, if food does not look good and taste good, you are not going to want to eat it day in and day out. The goal of overhauling your personal eating patterns should not be simply to lose a few pounds. It will be far easier to maintain your improved, healthier lifestyle if you view it as a whole new way of eating that you can and want to maintain without feeling deprived or cheated.

Modifying Recipes

Recipe modification is one of the simplest ways to introduce good nutritional cooking practices into your repertoire of dishes. You will soon find

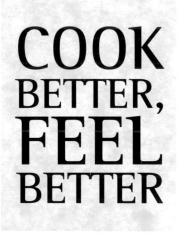

COOK BETTER, FEEL BETTER

The following suggestions can help introduce healthy cooking practices into any cooking style, whether you are preparing meals for a young family or for just yourself, whether you are a strict vegetarian or are a confirmed "meat-and-potato" person. You

will undoubtedly begin to see a change for the better on your plate and in your overall well-being as healthy practices start to become the rule.

• **First look at what you are currently eating and write down all the foods and drinks you eat over three days.** Then look at one of the food models and compare your diet with it. Which groups do you eat too much of, and which too little?

Decide on the changes needed and introduce them gradually. You don't need to do it all at once, but set realistic goals and try to achieve them. You are more likely to succeed by making adjustments fairly gradually.

• **Place a greater emphasis on grains, legumes, vegetables and fruits, rather than relying on meats, fish or poultry as the "center of the plate".** Many ethnic cuisines popular today have traditionally relied on this practice, and it ensures the inclusion of plenty of complex carbohydrates including fiber, vitamins and minerals. Top a steaming mound of couscous with a savory vegetable stew, for example, or serve curries over a steaming rice pilaf. Polenta or grits can be broiled (grilled) and topped with ragouts of mushrooms or eggplant (aubergine). If you are serving animal-based

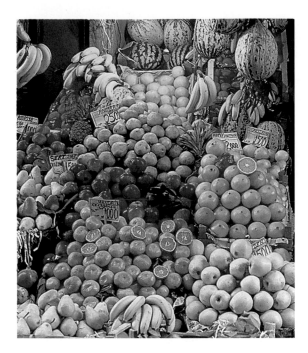

▲ Fresh produce provides a wide selection of nutrients essential for good health.

many ways to modify and adapt your current, comfortable cooking style to meet your new expectations for overall health and well-being through better eating. You can make some simple adaptations by broiling (grilling) a piece of chicken instead of sautéing it or replacing a fatty cut of meat with a leaner one.

Stuff vegetables with mixtures of rice and vegetables rather than meats. Replace the ricotta and eggs in your lasagne filling with steamed spinach and mushrooms seasoned with plenty of herbs and garlic.

Purchasing for Nutrition

Making the right choices at the market can make a great difference to your diet. It is also the best means of assuring yourself all the richest sources of the nutrients. The following suggestions are a good way to begin.

PRODUCE

If you have the time, space and inclination, there is no better way to assure yourself of fresh vegetables, fruits and herbs than to grow them yourself. Even if you live in an apartment, you can grow some varieties in window boxes or as potted plants. Failing that, search out greengrocers, farmer's markets, orchards and farms that offer cooperative growing programs or

foods (which are excellent sources of iron and zinc), use smaller portions.

- **Use monounsaturated or polyunsaturated fats and oils whenever possible and reduce the use of saturated fats.** Not only does the total amount of fat in your diet have an effect on your overall health, but the kind of fats and oils you use also play a role. If a recipe calls for butter, lard or shortening (margarine), which are all saturated fats, you may be able to replace those ingredients with an oil such as olive, canola (rapeseed), corn, safflower or peanut. Use the smallest possible amount of these oils when you sauté or pan-fry because even though they are less saturated than butter or shortening, they are still high in calories.

- **Use high-calorie and high-fat foods (eggs, cream, butter, cheeses and refined sugars) sparingly.** This step often presents the greatest challenge to anyone who has grown accustomed to relying on rich foods to act as the major carriers of flavor on a plate.

  Cutting calories should always include cutting fats. Cream, cheese, butter and oils add more calories, weight for weight, than other foods. When you do add them to a dish, use them sparingly. Use smaller quantities of strongly flavored cheese or grate a little cheese over your pasta, in place of a cheese sauce. Use low-fat versions of dairy products when you can and substitute low-fat yogurt or fromage frais for cream in soups and flans.

- **Learn a variety of seasoning and flavoring techniques to help reduce a reliance on salt.** Salt is relied upon as a seasoning and flavor enhancer in many dishes. If you are used to seasoning foods generously with salt, you may need to take the time to measure salt, instead of adding it "to taste". Gradually, you will lose your tolerance for lots of salt.

19

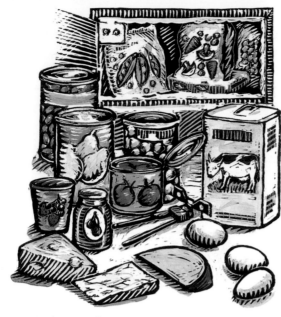

substitutes. Canned tomatoes, beans and other fruits and vegetables are also good choices. Be sure to read the labels and opt for reduced-sodium, reduced-sugar or lower-calorie versions whenever you can.

DAIRY PRODUCTS

Instead of whole milk products, look for products prepared with skim milk or part-skim milk. Reduced-fat types of yogurt, cheeses and sour cream are widely available.

MEATS, POULTRY AND FISH

Concerns about the quality and wholesomeness of meats, fish and poultry seem to grow each day. Many people have grown increasingly wary about where they purchase these items, as well as how often they eat them, if they still include them in their diets. If you follow the suggestions of eating pyramids, your overall consumption of animal foods will drop and be in smaller quantities. In that case, it might make sense to invest a little extra time and effort in finding the best possible purveyor and looking for organically raised meats.

"pick-your-own" operations. Stores that feature natural or organic foods are also a good source of high-quality produce.

The fresher the produce is, the better choice it is. When fresh fruits and vegetables are difficult to find or are too expensive, frozen or even canned versions are frequently good

---

There are many other ways to add flavor to foods. Wines, vinegars, citrus juices, spices, fresh herbs and low-sodium soy sauces can all be used.

Some ingredients, such as capers, bacon, olives, hard grating cheeses, processed and canned or frozen foods, may already be high in salt or sodium. Choose low-sodium options when you can and/or cut back on the added salt if you are including these types of ingredients.

- **Know what a "healthy" standard serving of the foods you eat looks like.**
Portion control is one of the most effective ways to help improve the nutritional

profile of a meal. By removing the skin from chicken, trimming visible meat fat and omitting the cream, you will considerably reduce the amount of fat, cholesterol and calories. Reduce portion sizes of meat, fish, poultry, dairy foods and fatty foods.

Increase portions of fruits and vegetables and make starchy foods—whether bread, potatoes, grains or pasta—the bulk of the meal. This will increase antioxidant vitamins, minerals and fiber levels.

- **Prepare and cook all foods carefully to preserve their nutritional value, flavor, texture and appeal.**

Chopping foods early, overcooking them, keeping them warm for too long or stewing them in water can destroy or cause essential nutrients to leach out. It will also affect the taste. Match the cooking method you select to the food you are preparing. Use methods that do not introduce additional fats and oils whenever possible. Broiling (grilling), dry roasting, boiling, microwave cooking and steaming are good examples.

Cook foods as close as possible to the time you plan to serve them. This will minimize nutrient loss, as well as ensure that the food is at its best when you put it on the table.

Some cuts of meats and poultry are naturally leaner than others. Skinless chicken breast, for instance, is a leaner option than chicken thighs with the skin on. Beef that has relatively little marbling or that has been trimmed to remove all visible fat is also a good choice.

White fish such as sole or flounder are typically lower in calories and fat than oily fish such as salmon, trout or mackerel. However, experts feel that oily fish are beneficial to one's health and should be included in the diet once or twice a week.

Smoked, cured or processed meats such as bacon or sausage can still be used, as long as you exercise care and moderation. Look for reduced-sodium-and-fat versions. Serve them once or twice a month or in very small amounts a few times a week, if you like.

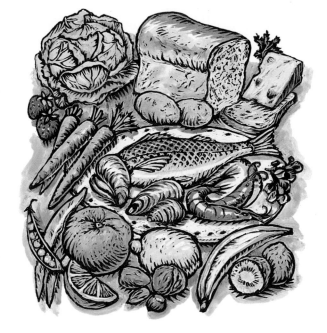

GRAINS AND CEREALS

Rice, millet, corn and other grains are widely available. Try other grains, too, and do not forget that pasta, potatoes, bread and noodles are all starchy nutritious foods—just remember not to add too much high-fat sauces and spreads.

Look for whole-grain or minimally processed versions of these items for the best nutritional value. They often contain a greater quantity of vitamins, minerals and fiber than refined versions.

- **Select foods that can do the most to help you meet your personal goals.** The foods you eat affect your sense of well-being in many ways. Pay attention to which foods make you feel vibrant and alive and which ones make you feel de-energized. Use the various charts and tables in this and other books to find the specific foods that offer the greatest nutritional benefit. If weight loss is part of your overall plan to feel better, choose foods with a high vitamin and mineral content but with few calories provided by fat.

  In general, the closer a food is to its natural state, the higher its nutritional value. Locally picked fruits and vegetables, for example, do not travel as far or as long to get to the market, which means that they will retain more of their nutrients than those that have been picked for a few days. Whole grains are a better source of a wider variety of nutrients than polished, refined or quick-cooking varieties.

- **Make your diet fit in with your lifestyle.** If you need to use a few processed foods, select low-fat versions or limit the number of times a week you consume them. Processed foods can be useful and the fact that they are processed doesn't necessarily mean they are not nutritious.

Frozen vegetables often contain more vitamins than so-called "fresh" ones, but if salt, sugar and fat have been added, the food may not fit in with your nutritional goals. Be sure to read any nutritional information on the label. Make comparisons to be sure that you are getting the most flavor, the best quality and the least unwanted additives possible.

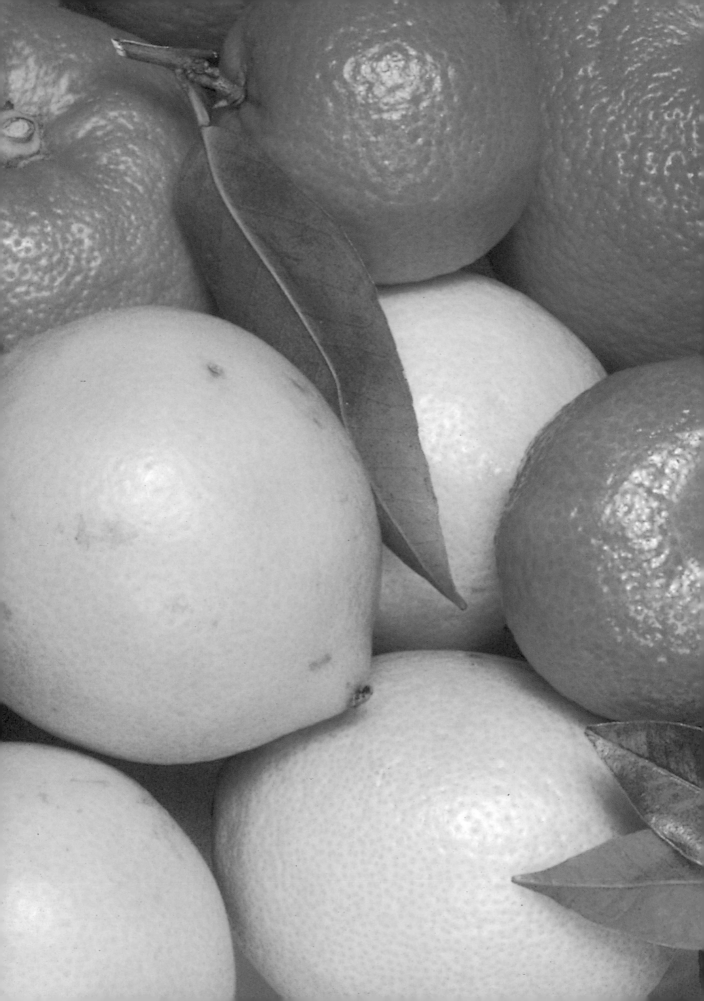

STAYING WELL WITH FOOD

What we eat or don't eat has a tremendous bearing on our health. Staying well with food is not just about using food as a neccssity and an enjoyment. It is about using food as a tool to fend off or even treat the common diseases and conditions that ail us.

Staying Well with Food

If you want to look and feel your best, you need to supply your body with all the appropriate fuel: a diet providing the right balance of nutrients, plenty of exercise, sufficient sleep and a strategy for dealing with stress. However, even with the best of intentions, you can still become worn-out and run-down, it is useful to know that many common conditions can be eased or prevented by the food we eat.

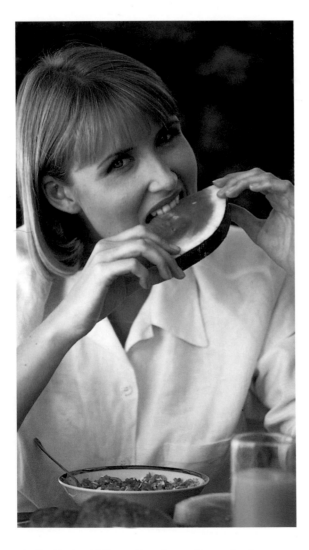

▲ *Eating healthily and staying well are closely linked. The food you eat has a large impact on whether you keep healthy or succumb to disease.*

Although we should always seek medical advice in the event of illness, this does not mean that our well-being is entirely in the hands of others. In Western cultures we all too easily relinquish rights over our own bodies and need to relearn how to control our own health and well-being. You live in your own body and should learn to recognize what it is telling you. Take the time to notice when you are feeling particularly well. What foods have you been eating? Which foods have you been avoiding? What kinds and amounts of exercise make up your daily routine? What is your emotional state? How well are you sleeping?

In a similar vein, pay attention to what your body is saying when you are not well. Has your regular routine been disrupted by something? Your physical environment can often offer clues. Have you changed an eating, exercise or sleeping routine? Have your relationships come under attack? Is the weather unusual in some way? Are you under an increased amount of stress? If you can begin to know how the answers to these questions affect your health, you are well on the way to becoming more in tune with your body. Realizing what makes your body tick means understanding how you can help to keep it in good health.

Remember that the lifestyle that works best for your own health may be totally foreign to others. Sleep needs, for instance, vary greatly

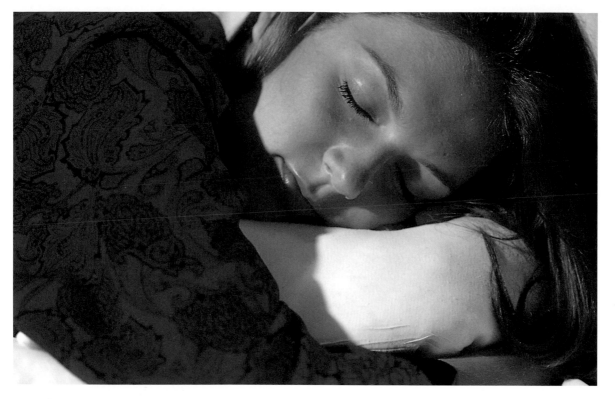

▲ *Late nights are sometimes inevitable, but getting the sleep your body needs is vital.*

from individual to individual. Don't berate yourself if you need nine or ten hours sleep each night to function well during the day. Conversely, don't crow if you can thrive on a high-stress lifestyle with fast food and little sleep. Surviving such a lifestyle depends on a whole host of circumstances individual to you, and a high-risk strategy that works for you today may turn against you tomorrow. It's worth remembering that nobody can abuse his or her body without paying for it in the long run. Whatever your current state of body and mind, looking after your health now will pay off in the future.

The information that follows in this section deals specifically with the dietary aspects of health and disease—explaining how the diet you eat can affect both your short- and long-term health. It is applicable whether you are bursting with health or less than well because it explains how nutrition affects the functioning of important body systems both in sickness and in health. This section also describes which groups of people may have extra nutritional needs and how these needs can be met. For example, the elderly may have reduced appetites but increased nutrient needs, so the concentration of highly

nutritious foods in their diets needs to be high. Similarly, pregnant women require extra nutrients to meet the needs of developing fetuses. Children, too, have different dietary needs, including higher fat requirements than adults in the fast-developing years from birth to the age of five.

Of course, the information offered in the following pages is in no way meant to replace the suggestions, advice and guidelines of trained health professionals. If you are experiencing a specific condition that does not respond quickly to some of the commonsense dietary measures suggested, it is time to take medical advice. And remember: regardless of which health practice or system you subscribe to, self-medication, even with harmless substances, can be counter-productive. On the other hand, eating an appropriate healthy diet can only make you feel fitter. Food provides the energy and nutrients to heal and restore and, combined with other healthy lifestyle practices, is the ultimate weapon in ensuring good health.

Eating better really can make you feel a hundred times better. No wonder the philosopher Aristotle said, "Let food be your medicine and medicine be your food."

133

General Health and Well-Being

Health is more than just the absence of illness; it's about feeling fit and mentally alert, having lots of energy and looking good. Maintaining a healthy weight, altering your diet to accommodate your changing lifestyle, and understanding the impact of diet on your appearance will all help in improving your general well-being. Certain foods will particularly help towards a fitter and healthier you.

The Balance of Good Health

As this book has already explained, one of the keys to maintaining the body is to provide it with all of the nutrients we know it needs by adopting a diet built around a good variety of the following types of food:

- Bread, cereals and potatoes—base meals on them.
- Fruit and vegetables—aim for five servings daily.
- Meat, fish and alternatives (legumes, nuts, eggs)—two to three servings daily.

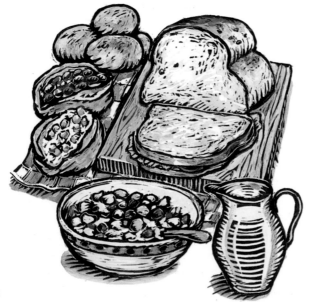

- Milk and dairy foods (preferably reduced fat)—eat two to three servings daily.
- Fatty and sugary foods—eat in small amounts.

There is also growing evidence that alcoholic beverages taken in moderation (especially one to two glasses of red wine daily) can play a role in maintaining healthy blood cholesterol levels.

In many industrialized societies it has become increasingly difficult to avoid highly processed foods. However, avoiding such items as excess sodium (salt), sugar and fat is important. Too much sugar and fat can lead to problems such as excess weight and obesity, heart disease and diabetes. Excess salt has been shown to contribute to high blood pressure, which is a precursor to heart disease. And more than one-third of cancers could be prevented by reducing high fat, highly processed foods in the diet and replacing them with more starchy, high-fiber foods such as fruit and vegetables.

Particular Needs

At certain times our lifestyles may require us to pay more attention to what we eat in order to meet our nutritional needs. Women have increased requirements during pregnancy and lactation, and young children and the elderly also have special nutritional needs. People who smoke

SUPER FOODS FOR GENERAL GOOD HEALTH		
FOOD	**RICH IN**	**GOOD FOR**
Carrots	Beta-carotene	Mopping up harmful free radicals that damage cells
Cabbage family	Gluco-sinolates	Fighting cancer
Citrus fruits	Vitamin C	Boosting immune system
Red wine	Flavonoids	Reducing the risk of heart disease
Soy	Phyto-estrogens	Speeding estrogen metabolism—possibly reducing breast cancer risk
Onions and garlic	Sulfur compounds	Boosting immune function, fighting cancer and heart disease
Oily fish	Omega-3 fatty acids	Improving blood flow; easing joint pain
Oysters	Zinc	Healthy immune and reproductive systems
Oats and beans	Soluble fiber	Maintaining healthy cholesterol levels
Brazil nuts	Selenium	Reducing cancer risk
Wheat germ	Vitamin E	Lowering heart disease risk
Yogurt	Friendly bacteria	Helping maintain a healthy digestive system
Liver	Vitamin B_{12} and iron	Preventing anemia
Olive oil	Mono-unsaturated fats	Maintaining a healthy cholesterol balance

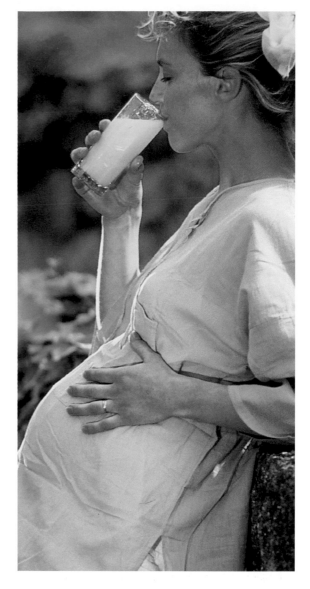

▲ *Pregnancy is a time to take special care of your diet. It is now known that a mother's nutrition can have far-reaching effects on her child's health.*

PREGNANCY

Pregnancy makes heavy demands on a woman's body, but most pregnant women can satisfy their needs and those of their growing fetus by eating a well-chosen diet that follows general healthy eating guidelines. The concept of "eating for two" is a well-worn excuse for eating excessively and gaining too much weight. In fact, for women who are not underweight at the beginning of their pregnancy, calorie requirements are not increased until the last three months, when up to 200 extra calories per day (equivalent to two to three slices of bread) may be required for the growing baby.

rob their bodies of valuable nutrients that need to be replaced, and highly active people also have greater nutritional needs. Vegetarians and vegans may need to plan their diets more carefully to ensure they achieve adequate nutrient intake.

Before Conception

When trying to conceive, it is important that both partners eat a healthy diet and avoid drinking too much alcohol as this can adversely affect fertility. Research has proven that the B vitamin folic acid can reduce the risk of a baby being born with spina bifida or other similar birth defects, so foods rich in folic acid—such as green leafy vegetables, fortified breakfast cereals and potatoes—should be eaten regularly. In addition, all women should take 400 micrograms (mcg) of folic acid daily from before conception until 12 weeks into pregnancy.

Vitamins and Minerals

Needs for certain B complex vitamins (required for energy release) are increased in pregnancy, but including adequate amounts of grains, fish, milk and lean meat in the diet should cover these needs. Vitamin C requirements are also increased, but these can easily be met by eating citrus fruit every day. A dietary supply of vitamin D (which can also be supplied through sunlight) is essential in pregnancy to aid calcium absorption and the development of strong bones. This can be acquired by eating eggs (well-cooked), butter and especially canned fish. Vitamin A also needs to be increased by eating deep orange fruits and vegetables (such as apricots, peaches, carrots and pumpkin), dairy products or eggs. Liver is an extremely rich source of vitamin A, but it is not recommended in pregnancy because very large levels of the vitamin can harm the fetus.

Experts are divided about whether the need for iron is increased during pregnancy. The mineral is vital for creating the fetus's blood supply, and, if intakes are insufficient, the mother can become anemic. In the U.S. it is recommended that all women take an iron supplement during pregnancy, but in the U.K. it is generally felt that natural increases in the efficiency of iron absorption can cover the extra needs.

Whether your doctor advises you to take iron supplements or not, it is important to ensure an adequate dietary supply of the mineral. Good iron sources are red meat and liver, dark-green vegetables such as spinach and cabbage, dried fruit and fortified breakfast cereals (also see *Iron*, p. 120).

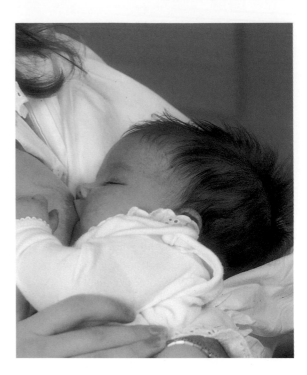

▲ *Breast milk is definitely best for a baby as long as the mother is healthy. Producing milk takes a lot of nutrients. This means that breast-feeding women need to pay special attention to their diet.*

EATING FOR PREGNANCY		
EAT PLENTY OF	**EAT LESS OF**	**AVOID**
Dairy foods	Fatty, sugary foods	Liver
Fish	Salt	Blue-vein, soft
Green leafy	Alcohol (no more	unpasteurized
vegetables	than a small glass	and mold-
Whole-grain cereals	of wine a day)	ripened cheeses
Fruit		

Pregnant women should ensure a good intake of calcium from dairy foods such as cheese, milk and yogurt. However, mold-ripened cheeses, such as Camembert, Brie, blue-veined and soft unpasteurized goat and sheep cheeses, should be avoided due to the risk of listeria infection.

Oily Fish

Scientists have found that omega-3 fatty acids present in oily fish, such as tuna, mackerel and sardines, are essential to early development of the fetal nervous system. Eating two or three portions a week of oily fish may be important for ensuring optimal brain development in the fetus.

BREAST-FEEDING WOMEN

Eating healthily is more important than ever after your child has been born. During breast-feeding, there are increased energy and protein requirements, as well as higher needs for many vitamins and minerals. Mostly these needs can be met by eating around 500 extra calories a day while adhering to healthy eating principles. As there are so many increased nutritional requirements during lactation, empty calories such as sugary foods should be avoided as much as possible. A modest multivitamin and mineral supplement may be a nutritional safeguard for busy breast-feeding mothers.

THE ELDERLY

Older people may experience a reduction in appetite or might find it more difficult to prepare and enjoy meals. Official tables often suggest that older people actually require fewer vitamins and minerals due to decreased energy expenditure, but in practice, requirements may be greater because of less efficient absorption. In particular, there is strong evidence that aging increases the requirements for vitamin D—needed for strong bones and the prevention of hip fractures—and certain B vitamins, which are particularly

important for brain function and energy release. Liver is an excellent food that includes both these nutrients and should ideally be eaten by the elderly once a week.

It is not always easy for older people to change the dietary habits of a lifetime, but the following practices can easily be incorporated:

- Drinking a glass of fruit juice every day
- Starting the day with high-fiber, whole-grain breakfast cereal
- Eating meat or fish once a day
- Eating one or two servings of vegetables every day
- Taking a drink made with hot milk before bed (one that does not contain caffeine)

Older people should be encouraged to keep an emergency food supply for times of illness or bad weather. Some nutritious suggestions include canned soup, dried fruit, long-life milk, instant mashed potatoes, canned fish, breakfast cereals, cartons of fruit juice and crispbread or crackers.

▼ *Getting older doesn't mean you can give up eating healthily; in fact, a good diet can be the key to keeping fit and healthy until a ripe old age. However, elderly people may have special nutritional needs.*

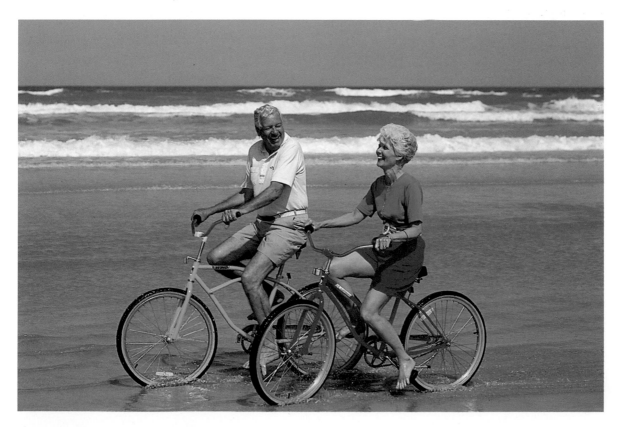

CHILDREN AND TEENAGERS

Preschool age children are developing rapidly and need to eat plenty of calories to support their growing bodies. Fat is a concentrated source of calories, and intake in preschoolers should not be restricted. Use full-fat dairy products for this age group, and avoid a very high-fiber diet as it may be too filling without supplying the right amount of calories. A combination of refined and whole grains is perfectly suitable, but avoid added bran or high-fiber breakfast cereals.

Recently, concerns have been expressed about low iron levels in the diets of both teenagers and younger children. Iron deficiency is associated with lower IQ scores and poor concentration. Including more lean red meat in the diet can help keep iron levels adequate and is especially important for preventing anemia in menstruating young females.

▼ *Children under five need full-fat foods to keep up their calorie intake. Dairy products are particularly important for developing bones and teeth.*

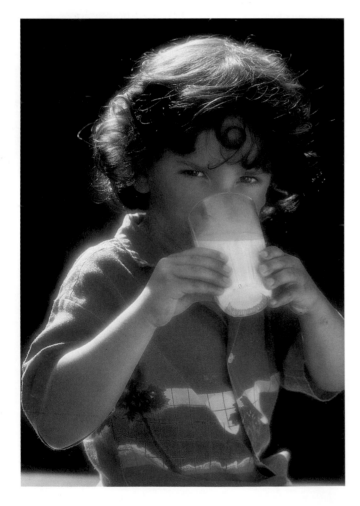

FOODS FOR PRESCHOOLERS	
EAT PLENTY OF	**EAT LESS OF**
Full-fat dairy products	High-fiber cereal, whole-grain
Red meat	breads and cereals
Fruit and vegetables	Reduced-fat products

SMOKERS

All smokers know the health risks they take. Each puff of smoke contains literally billions of free radicals—unstable molecules that attack and oxidize body cells—and the only way to stop the damage they cause is to quit completely.

In the meantime, smokers have increased nutritional needs, particularly for vitamin C and other nutritional anti-oxidants that offset the damaging effects of free radicals. Including a wide range of fresh fruits and vegetables in the diet is the best way to meet this increased anti-oxidant need. Most authorities say smokers need 80–100 extra milligrams of vitamin C a day just to keep their blood levels the same as nonsmokers. That is the amount contained in one large orange or about half a bell pepper.

ATHLETES

Keen athletes have a greater need for energy and a wide range of nutrients than sedentary individuals. In particular, athletes may need more B complex vitamins to aid energy release in cells and more anti-oxidant nutrients (vitamins C, E, selenium and beta-carotene) to mop up the rogue oxygen molecules produced by large amounts of aerobic exercise.

For athletes, carbohydrate foods, such as pasta, bread, rice and potatoes also assume greater importance. Eating these foods regularly helps build a supply of glycogen (stored energy) in the muscles, to be used for muscular activity when needed. Very large quantities of protein used to be hailed as the best way to enhance performance, but it is now known that loading the system with protein is not necessary. Strength and endurance athletes may need to increase their protein intake a little, and all athletes should ensure adequate dietary levels.

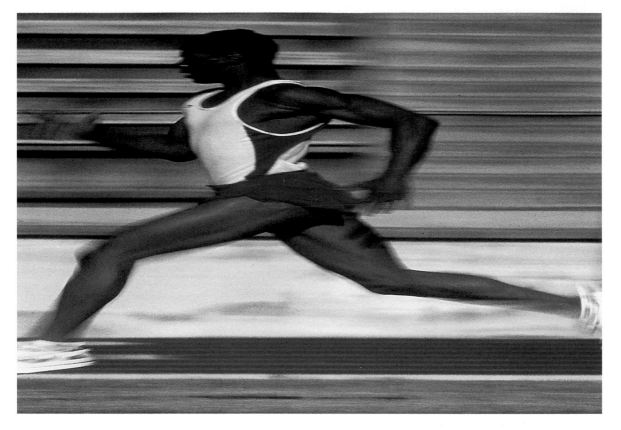

▲ *Athletes have increased nutritional needs and must eat more of certain foods for the very best performance.*

FOOD FOR ATHLETES	
EAT PLENTY OF	**EAT LESS OF**
Starchy carbohydrates, (e.g. pasta, bread, rice, potatoes)	Sugary foods
Fruit and vegetables	Foods with
Lean meat, poultry, fish	saturated fats

VEGETARIANS AND VEGANS

Most nutrients can be supplied adequately by a vegetarian diet, but intake of those which occur naturally only in animal food—such as vitamin D (for strong bones) and B_{12} (for a healthy nervous system)—may be marginal. Vitamin B_{12} can normally be obtained in sufficient amounts from dairy products, but vegans (who avoid dairy products and eggs) may need to take supplements and eat plenty of foods such as yeast extract, fortified cereals and soy milk. Vitamin D can be found in vegetable margarines and fortified breakfast cereals and can be made in sun-exposed skin.

Contrary to popular belief, most vegetarians and vegans actually consume adequate amounts of iron in their diets. However, absorption of the mineral from vegetable sources is very much poorer than from meat. In practice, vegetarians and vegans adapt to their diet by acquiring an increased ability to absorb iron, and their higher intake of vitamin C is also useful as this vitamin markedly enhances the uptake of iron from non-meat sources. However, vegetarians and vegans should avoid drinking tea with meals, as the tannins in the drink can have an adverse effect on iron absorption from plant sources.

Dietary intakes of bone-strengthening calcium are generally no lower in vegetarians than in meat eaters as both groups include dairy products in their diet. Vegans need to increase consumption of calcium-rich vegetable foods (for example broccoli and calcium-enriched soy milk) to compensate for the lack of dairy sources.

Another mineral of concern is iodine, which plays an important role in regulating metabolism. Vegetarians who regularly drink milk can obtain enough iodine, but vegans need to include fortified foods or seaweeds in their diets to ensure an adequate supply.

Weight Control

Most people can carry a little extra weight without too much detriment to their health. But people who are 20 percent over their healthy weight risk joint problems, high blood pressure and diabetes.

ARE YOU OVERWEIGHT?

The degree to which you are overweight can be determined by dividing your weight in kilograms (kg) by your height in meters squared (W ÷ H × H) to arrive at your Body Mass Index (BMI). If your calculated BMI is between 19 and 25, you are of an acceptable weight; between 25 and 30 indicates a degree of overweight; and over 30 indicates obesity. For example, a woman weighs 154 pounds (70 kg) and is 5 ft 2½ in (1.6 meters) tall. Her BMI = 70 kg ÷ (1.6 m × 1.6 m) = 27.3; so she is overweight.

To arrive at your BMI using pounds and inches, multiply your weight in pounds by 700. Divide the result by your height in inches squared. That is, BMI = (154 pounds × 700 ÷ 62.5 in × 62.5 in) = 27.5.

REGAINING CONTROL

Regaining control of your weight is simple in theory but hard in practice. There is no magic formula: Whether you lose or gain weight is a simple balancing act between the amount of energy (calories) ingested and the amount used up in daily activity and exercise. To lose weight, you need to reduce the number of calories you eat while ideally also increasing your amount of exercise.

Whatever your method of weight control, don't expect to lose more than 2 lb (1 kg) a week, and never go on crash diets as they inevitably lead to weight regain.

The following tips should also help in shedding the weight:

• **Always eat breakfast.** Studies show that people eat more calories in total if they skip the first meal of the day.

• **Use smaller plates.** Psychology plays a role in weight loss. Fool yourself into thinking you are eating a bigger meal by putting it on a smaller plate.

• **Graze, don't gorge.** Some people lose weight

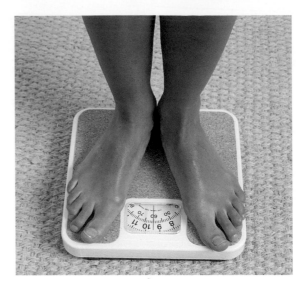

▲ *How you look is more important than what the scales say, but your weight is still important.*

better by spreading their calorie intake throughout the day and eating little and often. But you must be sure not to eat full meals *and* snacks!

• **Chew, chew, chew.** If you eat too quickly, your "fullness" sensors may not be able to react in time, and you could easily end up overeating. So take your time and chew every morsel well.

Looking and Feeling Good

Looking and feeling your best involve more than just being free from disease. They mean having loads of energy, clear skin and shiny hair. If this level of vitality eludes you, read on . . .

ENERGY AND STAMINA

Even if all we appear to do is sit at a computer all day, our hearts are pumping, synapses in the brain are firing repeatedly, our lungs are working and our muscles are holding us erect. In order to make it through the day without flagging, we need to ensure we have a good, steady source of energy for our bodies.

Carbohydrate foods are one of the best ways to raise our blood sugar (glucose) levels and to ensure that we are offering our bodies the energy they need. It was once thought that the speed at which a food raises blood sugar levels was determined by whether carbohydrates were simple (sugars) or complex (starches). But it is now believed to depend on the exact type of starch or sugar, the degree of processing it has received and how quickly it can be emptied from the stomach. In fact, complex carbohydrates such as bread and potatoes cause a quick blood glucose "high," while simple carbohydrates (sugars) such as fruit cause a slower response. Accompanying fat, fiber and protein, however, slow down the emptying of the stomach, so the quick "high" can be slowed down if, for example, you eat cheese with your bread or butter with your potato.

Use the following lists to help you choose foods that will keep your energy levels high throughout the day:

FOODS FOR ENERGY	
FOR A QUICK BOOST	**FOR A LONGER LIFT**
Bread, rice and potatoes	Beans and lentils
Raisins	Apples and cherries
Bananas	Yogurt
Orange juice	Whole-wheat pasta
Rice cakes	Oats
Cornflakes	Oranges
	Grapes

SKIN, HAIR AND NAILS

It is often said that you can see a person's state of health reflected in the condition of his or her skin, hair and nails, which are all affected by diet.

All tissues, including skin, hair and nails, are basically made up of protein and water, so including plenty of fluids and good sources of protein in the diet will help to keep them healthy. Small quantities of nuts, seeds and vegetable oils are also important as they contain essential fatty acids that keep the skin moisturized and waterproof. Zinc and vitamin A help combat dryness and pimples, and zinc also affects nail health. White flecks on the nails can indicate a deficiency of this important mineral.

Skin Aging

Anti-oxidant nutrients help to prevent the skin from aging prematurely. Some evidence suggests that the brightly colored carotenoid family of anti-oxidants may be particularly helpful in protecting the skin against sun damage. Flavonoids, found in the pithy parts of citrus fruits, may also be important in maintaining

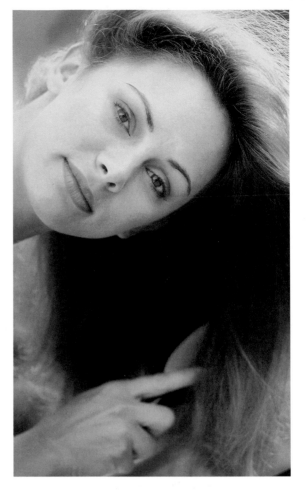

▲ *Skin, hair and nails reflect the state of your inner health and nutritional status.*

young-looking skin as they help maintain its firm collagen structure.

Hair Health

Healthy hair depends on various nutrients, including protein and B vitamins. An iron deficiency can lead to hair loss but is not usually the primary cause. Hormonal imbalance, stress and medication are often other important factors.

EATING FOR HEALTHY HAIR, SKIN AND NAILS	
EAT PLENTY OF	**EAT LESS OF**
Fruits and vegetables	Sugary foods
Nuts and seeds	Fatty foods
Fish, poultry and lean red meat	
Whole-grain bread and cereals	
AND DRINK	
Plenty of water	

Your Healthy Body

Your body has many different systems that, in times of good health, interrelate in perfect harmony. For example, the heart and lungs work together to oxygenate the body, while a part of the nervous system sends messages to the heart telling it to beat. The digestive system breaks down and digests foods to make them ready for absorption by the body, and hormones act on the digestive tract and affect the amount of certain minerals absorbed. The nervous system may also affect the immune system and hormone balance.

Although many factors can affect body systems (for example, smoking, stress, exercise, body weight), diet is also an important factor in determining how well these systems function. Understanding this can help to keep you well.

In this section we examine the different body systems and which foods or nutrients are important to help them function optimally. Understanding the delicate relationship between nutrition and body systems also helps if things go wrong.

▼ *Yogurt and garlic can help improve the balance of friendly bacteria in your digestive system. This can boost your resistance to intestinal infections.*

The Immune System

Eating a healthy, balanced diet will help ensure that your immune system functions optimally. Of course, having the perfect diet won't always stop you from catching a cold or coming down with flu, but it will mean you suffer less severely and bounce back more quickly from illness.

A diverse collection of cells, tissues and organs makes up the immune system. Skin is actually part of our immune system, acting as a barrier to dirt and bacteria. The mucous membranes in the nose, throat and respiratory passages act as primary protection against infectious micro-organisms, and we need vitamin A to keep these passages healthy.

If disease-causing bacteria are swallowed, stomach acid is designed to kill them, or friendly

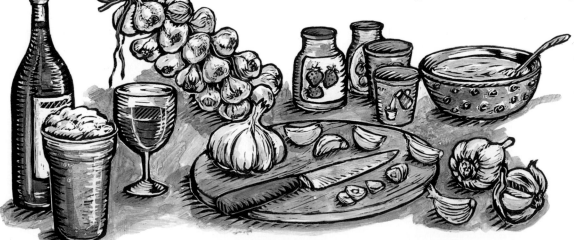

"bugs" in the intestines crowd them out. Yogurt, especially if it contains special cultures, can enhance the action of friendly gut flora against harmful bacteria. Garlic contains sulfur compounds, which also boost the immune system.

Inside the bloodstream, a whole range of immune-specific cells get to work to destroy any invaders that have passed the primary defenses. These require certain vitamins and minerals to work effectively, including vitamin C, B complex, vitamin E, zinc and selenium.

A little alcohol can boost the immune system, but always keep well within safe limits. Sufficient sleep relaxes the body and allows the immune system to rejuvenate, while moderate exercise stimulates the circulation, increasing the efficiency of immune cells. On the other hand, smoking and excess alcohol load the body with toxins that tax the immune system; excess fat makes immune cell circulation sluggish, and too much sugar can also affect immunity.

EATING FOR BETTER IMMUNITY	
EAT PLENTY OF	**EAT LESS OF**
Fruits and vegetables	Sugary foods
Yogurt	Fatty foods
Garlic	
Nuts, seeds and grains	
AND DRINK	
Orange juice	

The Bones and Joints

Strong, healthy skeletons are essential to carry us through life. Bones may seem like "dead" structures, but they are in fact made of living tissue, which is constantly being remodeled. Eating a calcium-rich diet helps maintain bone strength and is particularly important before the age of 30, when peak bone mass is achieved. Regular weight-bearing exercise (for example, walking, jogging, skipping) also encourages strong bones, as do other nutrients including vitamin D, zinc, magnesium and copper. High-fiber diets may reduce the absorption of minerals important for healthy bones, so it may be wise to avoid added bran.

Joints exist where two bones join together

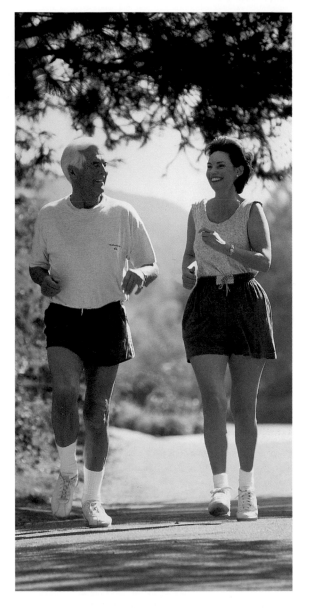

▲ *Keeping fit is essential to health. Movement of the joints through walking or jogging encourages strong bones—although care should be taken not to injure the joints.*

and, naturally, after many years of bending, walking and stretching, they can suffer from wear and tear. However, the cartilage and lubricating fluid surrounding the joints can be protected by consuming a diet rich in vitamin C—found in citrus fruits, bell peppers and blackcurrants—and the mineral manganese—found in foods such as whole-wheat bread, legumes, hazelnuts and tea. Inflammation around joints can be kept at bay by including oily fish in the diet and reducing the intake of saturated fats.

Muscles attach to the bones via tendons, and are made up predominantly of protein. With

143

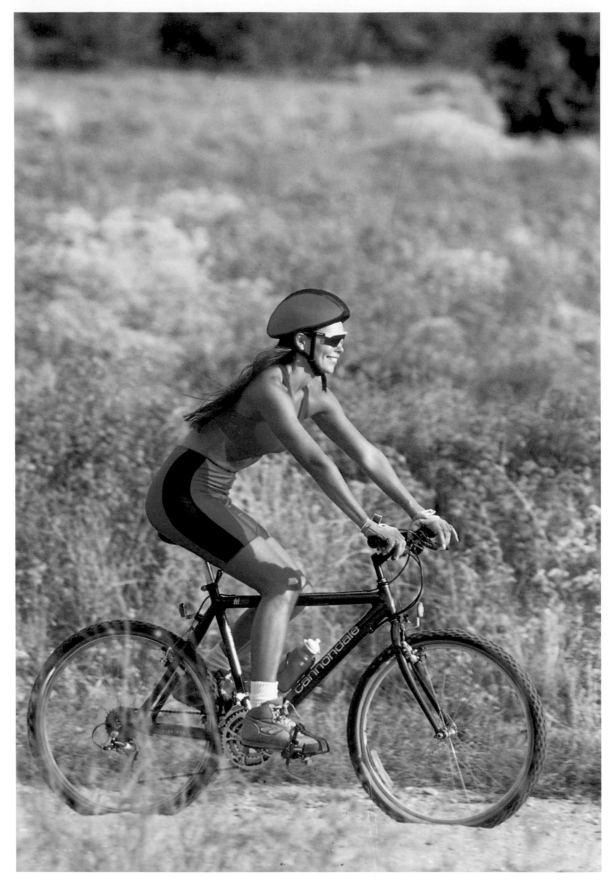

▲ *A healthy diet combined with regular exercise is the ideal combination for a strong heart and lungs.*

every movement, muscles are required to contract or relax; the energy for this process is supplied by carbohydrates. Calcium and magnesium are also essential for muscles to function correctly.

EATING FOR HEALTHY BONES AND JOINTS	
EAT PLENTY OF	**EAT LESS OF**
Reduced-fat dairy foods	Added bran
Oily fish, (especially canned fish with bones)	Saturated fats (fatty meats, cookies [biscuits], pastries, and so on)
Green vegetables	
Nuts, seeds and grains	

The Heart and Lungs

The heart circulates blood carrying oxygen and nutrients around the body. The left-hand side of the heart pumps oxygenated blood from the lungs to the tissues, and the right-hand side pumps low-oxygen blood back from the tissues to the lungs. To maintain a regular beat, the heart requires the right balance of minerals including potassium and magnesium. Aerobic exercise (exercise which utilizes oxygen) strengthens the heart muscle and helps it beat more efficiently. Being overweight and consuming too much saturated fat and salt tend to raise blood pressure and cholesterol—risk factors for heart disease. Diets rich in oats, fish oils, vitamin E and garlic are believed to reduce the risk of heart disease.

The lungs completely fill the thoracic cavity, and breathing is brought about by increasing and decreasing the size of this cavity. Pollutants such as cigarette smoke can markedly reduce the efficiency of the lungs. Antioxidant nutrients, such as vitamin C and beta-carotene help protect lung function.

EATING FOR A HEALTHY HEART AND LUNGS	
EAT PLENTY OF	**EAT LESS OF**
Fruit and vegetables	Salty foods
Garlic	Saturated fats (fatty meats, cookies [biscuits], pastries, and so on)
Oily fish	
Avocados, wheat germ, nuts and vegetable oils	
Oatmeal (porridge)	

The Reproductive System

Nutrition is important in maintaining a healthy reproductive system in both men and women. In particular, the mineral zinc is vital for maintaining fertility. This mineral is found in grains, meat and nuts and is particularly plentiful in oysters.

Antioxidants help maintain the integrity of male sperm, and some studies have shown that increasing the intake of vitamin E (found in avocados, wheat germ, nuts and vegetable oils) can increase the number of undamaged sperm and increase their mobility.

EATING FOR A HEALTHY REPRODUCTIVE SYSTEM	
EAT PLENTY OF	**EAT LESS OF**
Seafood (especially oysters)	Sugary foods
Citrus fruits	Foods with saturated fats
Avocados, wheat germ, nuts and vegetable oils	

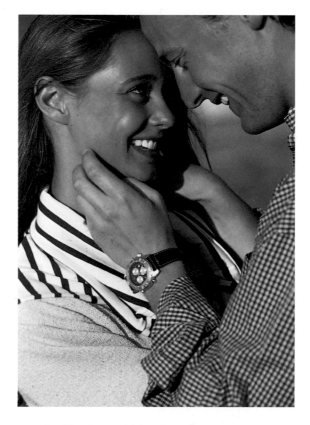

▲ *A healthy diet and lifestyle can enhance your love life and improve fertility.*

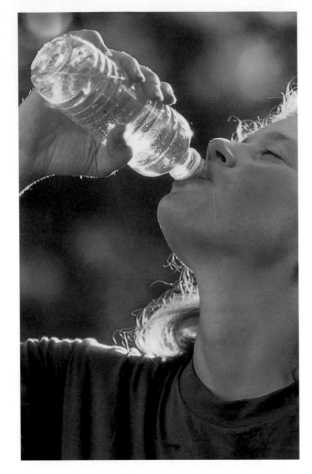

▲ Drinking plenty of fluid (around eight glasses of water every day) keeps our kidneys functioning correctly and removes toxins from the body.

EATING FOR HEALTHY DIGESTIVE AND URINARY SYSTEMS	
EAT PLENTY OF	**EAT LESS OF**
Whole-wheat bread, pasta and rice	Sugary foods
Fruits and vegetables	Saturated
Beans and legumes	fats
AND DRINK	
Plenty of water	

The Digestive and Urinary Systems

The digestive tract consists of the mouth, esophagus, stomach, small intestines and bowel (large intestines), and its purpose is to break down food into smaller and smaller parts, which are then absorbed by the body.

Fiber in foods such as fruit, vegetables and whole-grain cereals is very important for a healthy digestive system because it adds bulk to the feces and enables toxins to pass more quickly out of the body. Fiber also has the ability to bind small amounts of fat and cholesterol and remove them from the body.

Adequate fluids are necessary for the fiber to do its work as a bulking agent. Water is also vital for a healthy urinary system. It flushes toxins from the kidneys and reduces the risk of bladder infection.

The Nervous System and Hormones

The nervous system is made up of a very large number of nerve cells that transfer electrical messages from touch or pain sensors in the skin to the brain, and from the brain to the muscles. Electrical stimulation of nerves depends on the interchanges between various minerals in the body, particularly potassium (abundant in dried fruits and bananas) and sodium. Messages passing from nerve to nerve or from nerve to muscle do so via neurotransmitters, and good nutrition can ensure proper production of these chemical messengers. For example, one common neurotransmitter requires choline for its formation, and this is found plentifully in egg yolks, wheat germ, soy and liver. Other neurotransmitters require B vitamins to function properly.

Hormones also act as chemical messengers, but they originate in one part of the body and travel round the bloodstream to have an effect on another part. For example, parathyroid hormone is produced by a gland in the neck, but it acts on the digestive tract, stimulating the absorption of calcium. To maintain a healthy hormone balance, a wide range of nutrients is required.

EATING FOR A HEALTHY NERVOUS SYSTEM AND HORMONES	
EAT PLENTY OF	**EAT LESS OF**
Whole grains, whole-wheat bread and pasta, and brown rice	Highly refined and processed food
Lean meat, poulty, liver and eggs	
Dried fruits and bananas	
Fruits and vegetables	

Your Unhealthy Body

The body can all too easily become diseased, and when major body systems are attacked, the effects can be devastating (for example, the bones and joints in arthritis). The two commonest major illnesses that affect Western societies are heart disease and cancer. The good news is that in both cases, eating the proper diet can significantly reduce a person's risk of developing them.

Heart Disease

Poor dietary habits, lack of exercise and certain "lifestyle choices" have a great deal to do with how vigorously your blood flows, your heart beats and your entire circulatory system operates. Heredity plays a part, too; some families have histories of high blood pressure, raised cholesterol, heart attacks and strokes. To maintain the best overall cardiovascular health you need to adopt a diet that is high in fruits and vegetables (eat at least five portions a day) and low in saturated fats. Cut back on fatty red meats and learn to prefer meals based on fish. A vegetarian diet, as long as it is not heavy on fatty foods such as cheeses and eggs, may be a helpful choice for some people.

HIGH CHOLESTEROL

Cholesterol is a fatty substance made by the body and found in foods. As cholesterol deposits build up on the interior of arteries, the flow of blood is restricted and eventually blocked. The blockages prevent blood flow to the heart or brain and may lead to permanent damage and heart attacks or strokes (particularly for those with an inherited tendency towards high cholesterol levels). For most people, the amount of cholesterol consumed bears little relation to cholesterol levels in the bloodstream. This is because the liver can reduce its production of cholesterol in response to high levels ingested in food. What does raise blood cholesterol, however, is saturated fat: Avoid cookies (biscuits), cakes, cream, pastry and fatty meats. Increasing your intake of antioxidants in vegetables and fruits stops cholesterol from becoming oxidized, which is the precursor to narrowing of the arteries.

147

HIGH BLOOD PRESSURE (HYPERTENSION)

While very common, high blood pressure is undesirable because it can lead to heart attack or stroke if unchecked. Some individuals suffer from stress-induced high blood pressure; others suffer from it as a result of being overweight or having diets that are too high in sodium. There may also be an inherited tendency to have high blood pressure.

Help to keep your blood pressure normal by cutting down on salt in food. About 25 percent of our sodium comes from the salt we add at the table, so resist the temptation to shake before you taste. Processed and "fast" foods, however, are by far the biggest source of sodium in our diets. Try to eat less of these and to concentrate on potassium-rich foods instead, especially fruits and vegetables. Eating more oily fish and garlic and keeping your weight within normal limits will also help to keep blood pressure from rising.

Avoiding a Heart Attack

Following the dietary tips in the previous two subsections will do much to reduce your risk of suffering a heart attack. It is particularly beneficial to incorporate oily fish into your diet, as this provides important omega-3 fatty acids, which reduce the stickiness of the blood and improve its flow. Researchers believe that two or three servings a week will reduce the risk of heart attack. In people who already have a degree of heart disease, a daily 400 i.u. vitamin E supplement is also beneficial and may reduce the risk of a nonfatal heart attack by as much as 75 percent.

A pleasurable component of a diet that aims to reduce the risk of heart disease is red wine. The flavonoids it contains act as anti-oxidants and stop platelets in the blood clumping together. Try not to exceed two glasses a day.

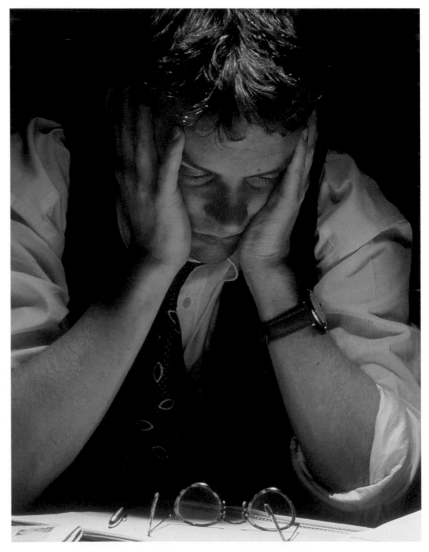

▶ *Stress is a major factor in raising blood pressure and increasing the risk of heart attack. A healthy diet will help offset some of the effects of stress, but you should take time to relax too.*

Cancer

Science is still working to unravel many mysteries associated with cancer. Hereditary factors mean some individuals are affected, while others are not. Cancers are typically slow to develop, so early detection and treatment are valuable in preventing death.

Environmental factors, such as toxins in polluted air, industrial wastes and radiation are thought to be linked with cancer. Smoking is by far the leading cause of lung cancer, and a stressful lifestyle may also be a factor in some forms of the disease.

You may not be able to change your environment or genetics, but you can stop smoking and change your diet. As many as 35 percent of cancers are diet related, so eating correctly is a very positive step in cutting your cancer risk. We still need to learn a lot about diet and cancer, but below are some known steps you can take to reduce your chances of contracting the disease:

1. Maintain a healthy body weight.
2. Moderate the amount of smoked, pickled and nitrate-cured foods you consume (bacon, ham, smoked fish, corned beef) as these contain carcinogens (cancer promoting agents). Avoid burnt foods for the same reason.
3. Limit your intake of all fats. This may be especially important for women with a history of breast cancer in their family.
4. Eat a variety of foods that are rich in fiber (apples, oranges, beets [beetroot], tomatoes, oats, wheat, rice, beans, carrots, celery, pasta and corn, for instance).
5. Concentrate on including five servings each day of fresh fruits and vegetables. These foods are typically high in fiber and anti-oxidants. If possible, try to choose foods that are organically grown.
6. Include foods rich in vitamins A and C such as carrots, spinach, sweet potatoes, peaches, apricots, strawberries, potatoes and all varieties of citrus fruit.
7. Eat at least one serving each day of vegetables in the cabbage family: red, green, savoy or other cabbages, plus kohlrabi, broccoli, cauliflower or Brussels sprouts.

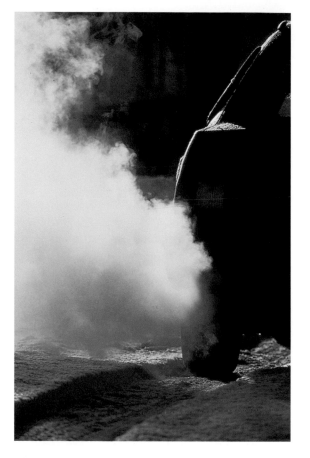

▲ *Cancer has many causes. Help protect yourself by eating a diet rich in antioxidant nutrients (such as fruit and vegetables).*

8. Women may want to increase their consumption of soy foods which some believe may reduce the risk of breast cancer.
9. Incorporate Brazil nuts in your diet. They are very rich in selenium, which is an anti-oxidant lacking in very many soils and which may protect against cancer.

Unfortunately, some of the treatments for cancer, such as chemotherapy and radiation, are very debilitating, sometimes producing unpleasant side effects. Vomiting, diarrhea, hair loss, weight loss and lack of appetite are common. Find foods that provide adequate nourishment in the most palatable form possible. Several small meals over the course of a day may be easier to handle than traditional large meals. Don't forget that food should be a pleasure, even while noting any possible interactions with medications being taken as part of the treatment.

Directory of Ailments

Ailments and health conditions, whether minor or chronic, can sometimes respond to special modifications in the diet. Of course, it is important to be diagnosed and treated medically too, but you will be surprised how healing the right nutrition can be.

The Immune System

FOOD ALLERGIES

Food allergies arise when the immune system reacts against a harmless food or other edible substances as if it were a poison. Food intolerance is less serious but still causes an upset stomach or vomiting.

Eat more fruits and vegetables for a healthy immune system.

Eat fewer foods that trigger the allergy or intolerance. Common culprits include milk, wheat, eggs, fish, shellfish, nuts, soybeans and additives.

COLDS

Everyone gets colds, but frequent suffering may indicate that the immune stem is overstressed.

Eat more zinc-rich foods, such as oysters, grains, meat and fish, or suck zinc lozenges which help stop cold viruses from replicating. Increase the intake of vitamin C (found in citrus fruits and juices) and colorful, beta-carotene-rich vegetables, both of which boost the immune system.

Eat less sugar and fat, which make the immune system sluggish.

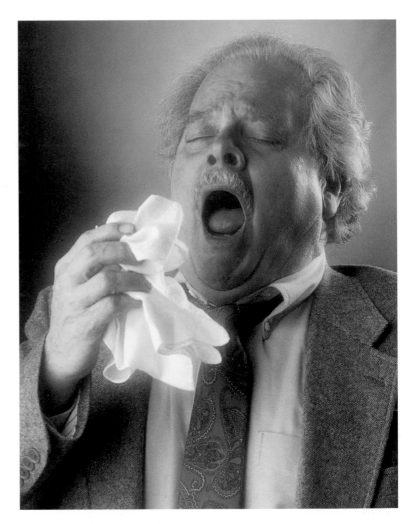

"ALLERGIC RHINITIS"

This is an allergy to pollen, molds, dust or animal dander, that causes a runny nose, itchy eyes and sneezing.

Eat more vitamin C-rich foods as they have an antihistamine effect on the symptoms.

▲ *Hay fever and colds are both signs that something is wrong with the immune system. Help protect yourself by increasing your intake of vitamin C.*

The Bones and Joints
ARTHRITIS
Rheumatoid arthritis is thought to be an illness of the immune system, whereas osteoarthritis is caused by wear and tear on joints. All types of arthritis result in pain, stiffness and inflammation of the joints.
Eat more oily fish, which encourages anti-inflammatory substances to be produced by the body, as well as fruits and vegetables rich in antioxidants. For osteoarthritis, eat more canned fish, which provides vitamin D for healthy bones.
Eat less fatty red meat and fewer full-fat dairy products and other sources of saturated fats, which may encourage inflammation in the body.

OSTEOPOROSIS
Osteoporosis is a bone-thinning disease that affects one in three women after menopause and an increasing number of elderly men.
Eat more calcium-rich foods including dairy products, broccoli and nuts.
Eat less salt and avoid heavy alcohol consumption—both leach calcium from the bones.

The Heart and Lungs
ASTHMA
Asthma causes constriction of the airways and (sometimes severe) difficulty in breathing. It is often associated with allergic conditions.
Eat more oily fish, which helps improve the balance of anti-inflammatory chemicals in the body. Increase your intake of antioxidant-rich fruits and vegetables, which help mop up harmful free radicals produced as part of the inflammatory process. Eating more magnesium (found in dark-green leafy vegetables) can also relax the airways. If your attacks are stress-related, step up your intake of legumes, grains and lean meat as they supply B vitamins vital for the nervous system.
Eat fewer foods that might provoke an attack. These vary from person to person but can include cows' milk, sulfite additives and wine.

POOR CIRCULATION
Poor circulation can manifest itself in cold hands and feet and may exacerbate symptoms of nerve damage in diabetics.
Eat more garlic and fish oils, which help reduce the stickiness of the blood and ease its flow. A supplement of the herb ginkgo biloba can also help.
Eat fewer saturated fats such as in fatty meats) as they can clog the blood vessels.

The Reproductive System
INFERTILITY
Infertility affects as many as one in six couples. If there is no physical cause, eating more of the right foods may help.
Eat more zinc-rich foods such as seafood, lean meat and grains, which help both the male and female reproductive systems including increasing sperm count. Increase the intake of vegetables and fruits and vitamin E-rich avocados, vegetable oils and nuts; these provide antioxidants to protect sperm function.

IMPOTENCE
Impotence can have many psychological causes but can also be affected by diet.
Eat more zinc-rich foods such as seafood, lean meat and grains, as these help to raise levels of the male sex hormone testosterone.
Drink less tea, coffee and colas as caffeine inhibits blood flow.

MENOPAUSAL PROBLEMS
Menopause can be a stressful time of life for women. As the levels of the hormone estrogen fall, the risk of brittle bones and heart disease increases. Symptoms include hot flushes, irritability, and dry skin.

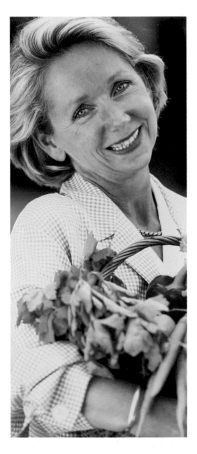

▲ *Women enter a new phase of life at menopause, but staying happy and healthy is within your reach with the right diet and lifestyle choices.*

Eat more low-fat dairy products and oily fish which provide, respectively, calcium and vitamin D for a healthy, strong skeleton. Increase the intake of wheat germ, vegetable oils, nuts, seeds and avocados, which are rich in vitamin E, for a healthy heart. **Drink less** tea, coffee and colas as caffeine can exacerbate hot flushes.

PREMENSTRUAL SYNDROME

Premenstrual syndrome (PMS) is a collection of physical and emotional symptoms suffered by many women in the days before a menstrual period.

Eat more regular meals rich in carbohydrates, vitamin B_6 and magnesium (good choices include bananas, dried fruits and nuts). These help keep blood sugar levels steady and feed the nervous system.

The Digestive and Urinary Systems

IRRITABLE BOWEL SYNDROME

As many as one in five people is affected by this condition. Symptoms, which arise because of abnormal spasms of the intestinal wall, include cramps, bloating, gas and alternating bowel movements (constipation and diarrhea).

Eat more foods high in fiber to encourage healthy digestive action. Regular, smaller meals can also help.

Eat fewer foods liable to cause flare-ups, including very hot or cold foods, caffeine and spicy foods. Avoid greasy meals as fat causes strong bowel spasms.

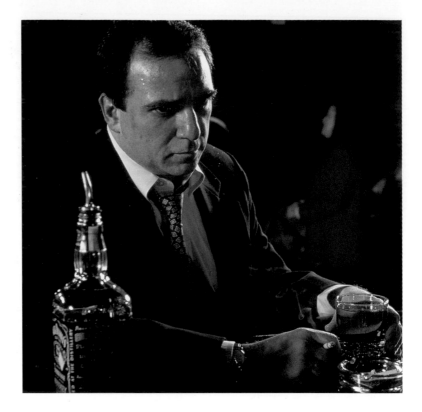

▲ *Stomach ulcers are exacerbated by alcohol, spicy foods and a high-stress lifestyle. Stop smoking and cut back on high risk foods.*

CYSTITIS

Cystitis is a painful bladder infection that causes a burning sensation during urination.

Eat more cranberries and drink cranberry juice. Cranberries contain a component that stops bacteria from adhering to the walls of the bladder. Drink plenty of water and fluids in general to help flush the bacteria from the system.

Eat fewer hot and spicy foods as they may exacerbate the condition.

ENLARGED PROSTATE

Lots of men develop enlarged prostates as they get older. Men who experience difficulty with urination should see a doctor, but eating more of the right foods can also help.

Eat more zinc-rich foods, for example, oysters, seafood, lean meat and grain to nourish the prostate. Increase the intake of processed tomato products (soup, pizza, baked beans), which supply an antioxidant called lycopene that may protect against prostate cancer. Supplements of the herb saw palmetto may also help.

ULCERS

Peptic (stomach) and duodenal ulcers have many causes, including bad diet, stress or infection with a bacteria called *helicobacter pylori*.

Eat more chili peppers! As long as you can tolerate them, chilies actually ease, ulcers.

Drink less milk—it may soothe an ulcer immediately but can lead to increased acidity of the stomach over the long term. Alcohol and spicy foods can also exacerbate stomach ulcers.

KIDNEY STONES

Kidney stones are caused by the painful crystalization of oxalic acid in the kidney.

Eat more calcium-rich foods such as dairy products. Contrary to popular opinion, these actually reduce the risk of developing kidney stones. Green vegetables, and grains that contain magnesium can also reduce the risk of stone formation. Drink plenty of water to dissolve the stone.

Eat fewer foods rich in oxalic acid, such as chocolate and spinach. Avoid high-dose vitamin C and calcium supplements if you are at high risk of kidney stones as these increase the level of calcium and oxalic acid passing through the kidney.

THRUSH

Thrush is caused by an excess growth of the *Candida albicans* yeast in the vagina—it causes itching and discharge. Thrush can also be present in the mouth where it causes a white growth.

Eat more live yogurt and garlic, which fight infection and encourage friendly bacteria to flourish.

Eat less sugar as it encourages the *Candida* yeast to grow.

The Nervous System
STRESS

A little stress can be very valuable, but too much can cause high blood pressure, muscular pains and depression.

Eat more Vitamin B rich foods, such as legumes, grains, lean meats and liver, which help to nourish the nervous system.

Eat less refined foods and avoid too much sugar as it depletes vitamin B_1 (thiamin).

DEPRESSION

Eat more carbohydrate-rich snacks, which raise the levels of the antidepressive chemical serotonin in the brain. Good choices include dried fruits, bananas and bread. Bananas and nuts include vitamin B_6, which can help PMS-related depression.

MIGRAINES

Migraines can have many causes, but certain foods are known to trigger them.

Eat more magnesium-rich foods, such as green vegetables, dried fruits, and grains, which help relax the muscles in the head.

Eat fewer trigger foods containing substances called tyramines, such as cheese, coffee and red wine.

General
FATIGUE

Factors ranging from too many late nights to hormonal changes or anemia may be responsible for fatigue.

Eat more lean red meat and liver to provide anemia-preventive iron and B vitamins. Vegetarians should increase their intake of dark-colored green vegetables.

Eat less refined sugar in sweet snacks as it can lead to fluctuating blood sugar levels.

SKIN DISORDERS

Skin disorders can range from occasional pimples to chronic psoriasis in which the skin reddens and flakes.

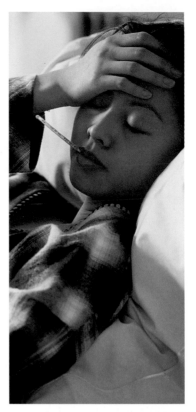

▲ *Fatigue can have many causes, so see your doctor. Eat a diet rich in iron and B vitamins. Avoid sugary foods that ultimately make you more tired.*

Eat more fruits and vegetables containing anti-oxidant vitamins and increase the intake of vitamin A (in foods such as liver and deep orange fruits and vegetables) and zinc to help improve acne. Eczema may respond to zinc and evening primrose oil. Oily fish may reduce inflammation in psoriasis.

Eat less full-fat dairy products and red meats.

CRAMP

Cramp is a condition in which muscles go into painful spasms.

Eat more calcium- and magnesium-rich foods (dairy products, grains, vegetables and nuts) which help muscles to function normally.

153

Glossary

Aerobic exercise Exercise such as walking or running that uses oxygen. After around 20 minutes of aerobic exercise, the body begins to burn fat significantly.

Amino acid Protein building block. There are eight essential amino acids that are not manufactured by the body and must be supplied by the diet.

Anaerobic exercise Energy expenditure that takes place without using oxygen. Anaerobic exercise includes sprinting, weight lifting and other short bursts of activity.

Antioxidant A dietary element or internally produced factor that protects body cells from becoming oxidized (rancid).

Atherosclerosis Narrowing of the arteries mainly through blockage with cholesterol and fats; a common precursor to angina or a heart attack.

Body Mass Index (BMI) A body mass measure that can be used to determine overweight or obesity; calculated by dividing your weight in kilograms by the square of your height in meters.

Bioavailability Ability of a nutrient to be available for use in the body. For example, iron from meat is more bioavailable than iron from vegetable sources.

Calorie The basic unit in which the energy value of food is measured.

Carbohydrate The body's preferred source of dietary energy, found in foods such as sugar, flour, potatoes and so on.

Carotenoids Important dietary antioxidants the most well-known of which is beta-carotene, also a precursor to vitamin A.

Cholesterol A fat-like substance made naturally by the liver. Although it is vital for the synthesis of certain hormones, in excess it can clog arteries; leading to heart disease.

Collagen Intercellular "cement" that binds together skin cells and other body structures including joint cartilage.

Fiber Non-digestible parts of food, such as, grains, vegetables and fruits, that improve digestive action and help to prevent constipation. Some types (soluble fiber) can be fermented in the digestive tract and may help to lower blood cholesterol levels.

Free radicals Chemically reactive molecules that play a part in oxidizing and damaging body cells and tissues.

Flavonoids Chemical components found especially in fruits, vegetables, red wine and tea. May act as protective antioxidants in the body.

Glycogen Storage form of carbohydrate found in muscles. It acts as a major source of energy for muscular activity.

Hydrogenation A chemical process that solidifies oils and effectively turns polyunsaturated fats into saturated fats.

Hypertension The medical term for high blood pressure. Hypertension is one of the major risk factors for heart disease.

Indispensable, or Essential, fatty acids Polyunsaturated fatty acids that can't be made in our bodies and have to be provided from dietary sources. Essential fatty acids maintain cell membranes and are needed to make important hormone-like substances that regulate many body functions such as the menstrual cycle, blood pressure and so on.

Legumes The edible seeds of any member of the pea family (including chickpeas, soybeans and lentils).

Listeria A bacteria which, while harmless to most people, can increase the risk of miscarriage in

EXPLANATIONS OF NUTRITIONAL SHORTHAND TERMS

Used in analysis charts on pages 24 –103 and 107–129

Ca	=	Calcium
CHO	=	Carbohydrate
CHOL	=	Cholesterol
Cu	=	Copper
Fe	=	Iron
Folat	=	Folic acid
I	=	Iodine
K	=	Potassium
Mg	=	Magnesium
MUFA	=	Monosaturated fat
Na	=	Sodium
NAeq	=	Niacin (vitamin B_3)
NSP	=	Fiber
P	=	Phosphorus
PRO	=	Protein
PUFA	=	Polyunsaturated fat
Se	=	Selenium
SFA	=	Saturated fats
Zn	=	Zinc

MEASUREMENT CONVERSION CHART

	U.S./U.K. Imperial		metric
Weight			
	1 ounce (oz)	=	28.35 grams (g)
	1 pound (lb)	=	453.6 grams (g)
	2.2 pounds (lb)	=	1 kilogram (kg)
Volume			
	1 fluid ounce (fl oz)	=	28.4 milliliters (ml)
	1.76 pints (pt)	=	1 liter (l)
	1 teaspoon (tsp)	=	5 milliliters (ml)
	1 tablespoon (tbl sp)	=	15 milliliters

Note: some U.S. and U.K. volume measurements differ; below are some typical examples:

		U.K. fluid ounces (fl oz.)	U.S. fluid ounces (fl oz.)
1 pint	=	20	16
1 quart	=	–	32
1 cup	=	10	8

pregnant women. May occur in blue-veined and unpasteurized soft cheeses, as well as patés.

Metabolism A term which describes all the chemical processes that take place in the body to keep it alive and functioning.

Microgram (mcg) A weight equivalent to one millionth of a gram (one thousandth of a milligram).

Micronutrient Vitamins and minerals that are essential to health but are needed by the body only in tiny amounts.

Milligram (mg) One-thousandth of a gram or 1,000 micrograms.

Monounsaturated fats Fatty acids (components of fat) which help to lower total cholesterol and improve the balance of cholesterol types in the blood. Olive oil is the richest source of monounsaturated fats.

Neurotransmitters Chemicals released in the brain and at the end of nerves to facilitate the passage of messages from one nerve to another.

Nonstarch poly-saccharides (NSPs) Technical term for fiber. The desirable intake of fiber measured as NSPs is $1/2$ ounce (18g) per day. (See fiber entry).

Omega-3 fatty acids A group of fatty acids that help to thin the blood and may protect against heart disease. A particularly rich source of these fatty acids are found in oily fish.

Organic meats These are meats from animals which have been raised on a nonchemical ethos, that is, they have not been treated with chemical growth stimulants, antibiotics or pesticides.

Oxalic acid A chemical that is toxic in high amounts and that in smaller amounts inhibits the body's absorption of minerals such as calcium and iron. Small amounts of the chemical are present in spinach, rhubarb and chocolate.

Polyunsaturated fats Fatty acids (components of fat) that help to lower total cholesterol but that are susceptible to becoming oxidized (rancid) in the body. Polyunsaturated fats are generally liquid at room temperature (for example, vegetable oil).

Protein Important dietary component that is vital for healthy skin, body tissue and muscles. Good sources are meat, fish and poultry.

Refined foods Foods such as white sugar, white flour and polished rice, all of which have been processed for better taste or more convenient use, usually with the result that some nutrients have been removed.

Saturated fats Fatty acids (components of fat) that contribute to raised blood cholesterol levels. Saturated fats have an inflexible chemical structure which makes them solid, even at room temperature (for example, butter).

Sodium Component of salt that may contribute to raised blood pressure.

Soluble fiber This is fiber that is partly broken down by bacteria in the intestines and may help in reducing cholesterol levels.

Starch (Complex carbohydrates) The major form in which energy is stored in plants. Bread, potatoes, pasta and rice are all good sources of starch.

Sulfites/Sulphites Compounds of sulfur used as additives in food. Mixed with acid, they form the gas sulfur dioxide used in wine making to kill yeast. In sensitive individuals, sulfites and sulfur dioxide may trigger asthma-type symptoms.

Tubers The underground stems of certain plants, such as the potato.

Toxic Poisonous or harmful to the body. A toxic compound is also described as a "toxin" and can be described as having "toxicity."

Vegetarian/Vegan A vegetarian is someone who does not eat the flesh of animals of fish. A vegan eats no animal products at all.

Index

Credits

Quarto would like to acknowledge and thank the following for providing pictures used in this book. While every effort has been made to acknowledge copyright holders we would like to apologize should there have been any omissions.

Ace Photo Agency p.137, p.138, p.139, p.141; **The Image Bank** p12, p.19, p.132, p.133, p.144, p.145, p.149, p.151, p.153; **Pictor International** p.136, p.146, p.148, p.150, p.152; **Powerstock** p.17, p.143; **Tony Stone Images** p.135.

All other photographs are the copyright of Quarto Publishing plc.

Quarto Publishing acknowledgements:
Senior Editor Gerrie Purcell
Text Editors Alison Leach, Trish Burgess
Senior Art Editor Penny Cobb, Catherine Shearman
Designer Neville Graham
Photographers Anna Hodgson, Paul Forrester, Laura Wickenden
Illustrator Valerie Hill
Picture Researcher Zoë Holtermann
Editorial Director Pippa Rubinstein
Art Director Moira Clinch